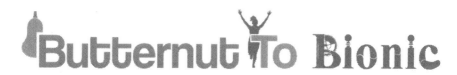

A Resource Guide for Hip Replacement Surgery

Tiffany Anderson, LMT, RMT, BS, CHES

Published by Glass Spider Publishing

www.glassspiderpublishing.com

ISBN 978-0-9979825-7-2

Library of Congress Control Number: 2017940052

Cover design by Jane Font

Edited by Jessica Beifuss

Author's Note: This book is not intended as a substitute for the medical advice of physicians. The reader should regularly consult a physician in matters relating to his/her health and particularly with respect to any symptoms that may require diagnosis or medical attention.

Publisher's Note: We endeavor to provide you with a book that is of the highest professional quality and free of printing errors. If the copy of the book you have purchased contains any printing errors, please contact us at info@glassspiderpublishing.com to arrange for a free replacement of this product.

TABLE OF CONTENTS

ACKNOWLEDGMENTS

This resource guide stewed and brewed for months in my mind and heart as I transformed into my new bionic self. With deep gratitude, there are a number of people that I would like to thank.

To my longtime physician and family practitioner, Dr. Leslie Peterson, who accompanied me on this medical mystery tour. Thank you for your gentleness and care, especially after reviewing my MRI and informing me that my hip joint had failed. To Brent Ottley, my acupuncturist extraordinaire and health confidant. Your expertise kept my pain at bay and your shoulder kindly accepted my tears along the way. To Dr. Jeremy McCandless, my brilliant surgeon. Without your time, expertise, and willingness to take on an uninsured patient, I'm not sure that I would have fared as well as I have. Thank you.

To my parents, who survived the stress and ordeal of experiencing their firstborn survive jaundice, liver failure, heart failure, extreme swelling, and arriving at dual-joint replacement. My dad, for staying by my side during each hospital stay. Thanks, Mom and Dad, I love you both. To my son, who joined me in fear and sat alone with me that first day home after hip replacement one. Thank you, kiddo, you are my light and I adore you. To my ex, Ike. Thank you for sharing part of a crazy ride with me, for wrestling with compression hose, taking care of my wounds, and for never telling me that my scars were ugly. To my clients, friends, coworkers, and medical staff who each helped along the way. Thank you.

Thank you to my long-term mentor, Terri Busch, and my massage therapist and Reiki practitioner, Allison Ottley. Two women I deeply admire who encouraged me to share my story and prepare this guide. To my writing coach, Nan Seymour, thank you for helping me polish chapters and maintain my flow. Thank you again to Brent Ottley and to Dr. Eugene Peay for providing valuable feedback on my manuscript. Finally, thank you to Glass Spider Publishing and *Utah Stories*—I found my publisher by reading an article about them in the latter. Without the professional guidance of Vince and Jane Font, Stephanie Simonson, Jessica Beifuss, and Cindy Jones, this final product would not exist.

Each and every one of you are amazing. Thank you.

Tiffany Anderson

IT ALL STARTED WHEN...

I looked into the mirror and saw yellow. Not cowardice—it was jaundice. My eyes, then my body, turned yellow—"butternut" is how my dad described it. Yellow as a butternut squash. From 2009 to 2011, I went from doctor to doctor and found no clear answers and no reason why I became sick. I didn't get better. Jaundice led to liver failure. Liver failure turned to heart failure, and my left leg began to swell. I rewrote my will and spent extra time with my family—especially my grown son. I traveled as much as I could afford and prepared for death at age 45.

Medications failed and diagnostic procedures nearly bankrupted me. For relief I turned to nutrition, meditation, prayer, Reiki, and acupuncture during what I believed were my final days. Through those methods, I found healing and pain management. Green drinks and a plant-based diet rejuvenated my liver and calmed my heart. My acupuncturist asked why no one had suggested an MRI. I didn't know either and got one.

Turned out I needed a hip replacement—and after surgery on my left side, I learned that I needed one on my right. Six weeks after receiving my second replacement, the damn thing slipped and failed due to a fracture, and we did the whole thing over again. We still don't know why all of this happened. What I know today is that I am managing my health and have a quality of life I am content with. I am no longer yellow—just a bit bionic.

My name is Tiffany Anderson and in 1996 I began my health career as a professional licensed massage therapist. I furthered my education to expand my scope of practice and improve my quality of life. My interest in health was driven early on from seeing relatives experience pain, disability, and disease from preventable conditions. My "aha" moment came at age 18 when I moved away from my parents' smoke-filled home and cured my childhood asthma. I realized that health isn't some elusive goal to chase; health is our natural state of being to nurture and maintain.

As my professional practice advanced, I began working in medical clinics and hospitals, at sporting events and in corporate settings. More and more of my clients were asking me questions about how to make long-lasting lifestyle changes and better manage their health. Continuing education credits to retain my massage license weren't enough; I needed more education to be of service to my clients and to myself. Not only did earning my bachelor of health education and promotion improve my professional standing, but that knowledge was invaluable when I personally experienced life-threatening illness leading to my need for hip replacements.

Artificial joints show up in people's lives under a variety of circumstances. If you're like me, you were baffled, a bit scared, and sad when diagnosed and informed that you needed joint replacement. Or perhaps you had been dealing with an injury or illness, and an artificial joint promised relief from an acute or long-term condition. Whatever the situation that led you to bionic status, you are among good company. In the United States alone, 400,000 people will receive a hip replacement every year[1]. In the past, this number has included celebrities such as Elizabeth Taylor, Jane Fonda, Katharine Hepburn (one of my idols), and Eddie Van Halen.

This book guides you through your hip replacement surgery by providing resources, suggestions, and checklists to help you prepare and adjust to what you might call your new normal. We want our hip replacements to stay with us for as long as possible, to avoid dislocation, and to enjoy as many activities and pursuits as we are able. On the pages that follow, I share personal insights, tools, and tips that supported me through a stressful time, three life-changing surgeries, and a dramatic lifestyle change.

Receiving artificial joints is a life-changing procedure. You feel different, move differently, and learn new ways of living. My goal is to avoid future surgeries and maintain the health and integrity of my current joints for the rest of my life. I believe I will succeed.

A resource that would have been beneficial for me during this transformative time was a support group or guide such as this for people receiving artificial joints. This resource was missing for me. To further fill that gap, I've designed a virtual space to connect and share our strengths, struggles, concerns, and successes. Fellow bionic buddies and others managing chronic conditions can find me online at www.andersontherapeutics.com. I offer coaching services, a wellness blog, plenty of free resources, tips, and tools to manage chronic pain. I use and promote three concepts to maintain good health, they are to *soothe, nourish, and rest*. These concepts are my foundation to live well and be well. I hope you find this information useful.

Yours in health,

Tiffany Anderson, LMT, RMT, BS, CHES

---

[1] Marchione M. Study: 2 percent of Americans have artificial hips, knees. New Jersey Herald website. Published March 12, 2014. Updated March 26, 2014. Accessed February 17, 2017.

CHAPTER 1
GATHERING SUPPORT—YOUR MEDICAL TEAM

*Believe in yourself. Someone has to make the first move.
—Found by Dr. Christiane Northrup on a Salada tea bag
during a conference on self-esteem (Women's Bodies,
Women's Wisdom).*

You've received the news—you need a hip replacement. Your feelings about this diagnosis may range from anger to sadness. I felt shock, fear, frustration, and confusion after learning that I needed a hip replacement. You will have questions, wonder what to expect, and even say, "Why me?"

I understand. This procedure isn't easy and requires your full attention for success. Each chapter of this book provides guidance, resources, and tips to help you through this challenge. What's first? It's time to make the first move and safely reach the destination as a healthy recipient. To begin, find a terrific medical team.

Consider the procedure you are embarking on as an extensive home improvement job. Your hip replacement is a rebuild and makeover of the original equipment you were born with. The contractor and crew are your medical team. You and your hip are the fixer-upper. Some people facing surgery may need only minimal contact with this crew and simply want the job completed with as few face-to-face discussions as possible. Others, like me, want every detail explained, only feeling safe and reassured with a close partnership from start to finish. Whatever your style and personality, we all have the same desire and that is a successful surgery and quick recovery.

11

Nearly two percent of Americans have either artificial hips or artificial knees. [2] More surgeries mean streamlined procedures, better implant products, and improved outcomes. However, receiving an artificial joint isn't without risk. Artificial joints have had recalls, and complications are, sadly, common. A large number of these complications before, during, and after surgery can be avoided. Prevention begins with you. The resources and tips outlined in this book can speed up your recovery, decrease your pain, and lengthen the life of your joint replacement. The first person to secure on your medical team is your surgeon.

Choose your surgeon carefully if you have choices available to you. If you're interested in a second opinion, you may want to speak to more than one surgeon. With an HMO, your family physician will refer you to a specific surgeon while a PPO allows you to visit any provider or physician as long as they are within your network. Check your individual plan and contact your insurance company to understand your benefits. I had no health insurance when I first learned that I needed an artificial hip, so I began my search a little unconventionally.

As an uninsured person, I was at a disadvantage while seeking qualified care, and understandably so—physicians and hospitals rightfully expect payment for services rendered. I happened upon an article in my local paper highlighting a free discussion conducted by an orthopedic surgeon. Coincidentally, the topic was arthritis and artificial joints. This miraculous find led me to my surgeon, Dr. Jeremy McCandless. After attending his presentation, Dr. McCandless graciously spent more than 30 minutes with me and my significant other, reviewing X-rays, and listening attentively to my story. He agreed to take me on as a patient.

CHOOSING A SURGEON

Besides you, the orthopedic surgeon is the head of the team. Check their credentials, inquire about their experience, and ask about surgeries they have performed. These aren't unreasonable requests. Have you ever needed extensive repair work for your vehicle or renovated a portion of your home? An estimate is drawn up based on the work required, a diagnostic is sometimes performed, and the outcome is discussed in detail. You want to know what is happening, how the changes will take place, and what it will cost. Your surgeon is basically rebuilding part of your leg! This rebuild is inside bone and within the largest muscles of your body. Ask if they have patient testimonials to give you an idea of who you are working with. Many insurance companies and doctors offer websites providing you with these details—it's okay to ask for reassurance and credibility.

State medical boards also offer information regarding physicians' backgrounds and whether they have been subject to any disciplinary actions. A detailed list can be found at the Federation of State Medical Board's website at www.docinfo.org.

The medical marketplace is very competitive, and a surgeon who is ethical and professional will want to reassure you, impress you, and earn your business. If you feel rushed or that your questions are disregarded or unanswered, shop around for a surgeon who is attentive, responsive, and respectful toward you. Your health and welfare are worth the time and effort.

WORKSHEET: QUESTIONS FOR YOUR SURGEON

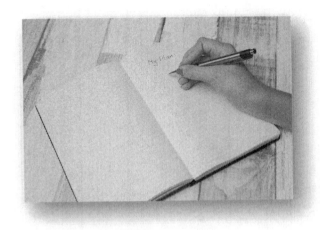

✓ Can you describe the procedure to me and tell me about any risks I need to be aware of?

✓ How can I better prepare for surgery?

✓ Are there any additional risks that I should be aware of?

✓ Will I have a posterior (through the back of the hip) or anterior (through the front of the hip) placement during surgery?

> Posterior placement is considered traditional and the most common approach. A posterior approach cuts through the buttocks to access the hip, requires a longer recovery time, and patients are at a higher risk for dislocation afterward. The anterior approach is less invasive and allows the surgeon to move muscles rather than cut through them. However, anterior placement isn't appropriate for some patients, requires special surgical equipment, and only certain surgeons are trained in this procedure. Depending on your situation, this decision will affect your recovery and how well you will be able to move long after you heal.

✓ Which type of device will you use for my hip replacement?

> I received a posterior placement using a ceramic-on-ceramic ball and socket device with titanium stem. There are five different types of devices used for hip implant in the United States, your surgeon uses factors specific to you and your health to determine which device is best for you.

✓ How long will the surgery take?

✓ How long will I be in the hospital?

✓ How soon will I be up and walking around after surgery?

✓ Will I be able to return home afterward or would I be better suited to transition to a rehabilitation center after I leave the hospital?

> Much of this decision will come post-op, though it is a good idea to talk about the possibilities well in advance and to check with your insurance company to learn if a rehab center is a covered expense.

✓ Will my current weight affect the surgery or recovery after?

> This is a touchy topic and one to take full responsibility with—**carrying an excess of five pounds can place 25 pounds of pressure on your joints**. This added pressure impacts every joint, not just the ones that are being operated on. Your doctor should encourage you to do your best to strive toward a healthy weight for your body type. Removing even a small amount of pressure on your joints helps you to move better, heal faster, and can *add years of use* to your new joint.

✓ Will I have stitches or staples? When do they come out?

✓ What type of medications will I be on and how long will I take them?

> Be prepared with a full list of your current medications with dosage amounts and how often you take them. Include any supplements, vitamins, herbs, homeopathic remedies, etc. Also, learn about different blood thinners and be sure to

discuss pain medications you will be prescribed prior to, during, and after surgery.

✓ Will any of my prescribed medications have side effects I need to be aware of?

✓ What limitations can I expect after surgery and for how long?

✓ Will I require physical therapy? If so, how long and how often?

✓ What type of assistive devices or home medical equipment will I need after surgery?

✓ Will I have physical therapy at home, in a rehabilitation facility, or will someone need to drive me to physical therapy?

Check with your insurance company. Is this a covered expense, and if so, how many visits are you allowed?

✓ When will I be able to drive a car?

This answer can depend on if you drive a manual or automatic transmission and which hip will be operated on. My left hip was the first to be operated on and I drove an automatic. This allowed me to drive after two weeks— getting in and out of a vehicle is tricky. To help you, the hospital physical therapy team may have a practice "vehicle" for you to get in and out of before leaving the hospital.

✓ How soon can I shower or bathe after surgery?

✓ When can I return to work?

✓ What about sex?

> My surgeon blushed a vibrant red at this question and wasn't quite prepared with an answer since I was much younger than most of his other patients. This is a valid question and one to consider *for adults of all ages*. Men and women will differ of course on how they are affected. I was told that intercourse was okay as soon as I felt well enough, simply to be aware of position limitations. Understand there is a great deal of post-op swelling, bruising, and significant pain—maintain open communication with your partner. This is a time for healing—if romance and love are alive, the physical aspect of your relationship will return in time.

✓ When will I see my surgeon after surgery and how many post-op visits can I expect?

> This answer will vary depending on your surgeon. I had built a strong relationship with my surgeon and saw him often. A friend of mine who received an anterior hip replacement saw her surgeon only once before surgery and was cared for by nurses and the physician assistant afterward. Understand that physicians manage patients differently.

✓ Add questions of your own in the space below.

THE REST OF THE MEDICAL TEAM

Once you've secured your surgeon, a number of preoperative appointments are necessary for X-rays, lab work, and assessments. These appointments provide your medical team with needed information to prepare for your surgery and lay the groundwork for changes ahead. Think of these appointments as the blueprint stage. The architect (your surgeon) needs to draft the plan to correct any faults, preparing for the removal of unwanted material, and adding new and improved parts.

The list below highlights additional players of your medical team. Establish a good relationship with each of them during this preparation stage. These professionals ideally want to gain your trust and assure you that your well-being is a priority. A strong medical team will ease your stress and instill you with confidence.

PATIENT (YOU!)—BE AN *ACTIVE* PARTICIPANT

An educated patient is one who is inquisitive and eager to learn; ask plenty of questions! By demonstrating this attitude, your medical caregivers learn that they are caring for a patient who is more likely to succeed during and after surgery.

A proactive approach also provides a sense of control during a frightening time. Take the extra step and learn about the procedure you are undertaking. Your surgeon may offer some educational material in-office, such as articles or brochures, describing joint replacement. Even if you are a bit squeamish, educate yourself as much as you can and read the materials provided to better prepare yourself. This isn't just getting some stitches, taking a prescription to treat bacteria, or even setting a broken bone, though all of those elements come into play with joint replacement. This is an invasive surgery. Be cautious when using a standard Google search. Below are some educational resources to guide you. And, unless you have a strong stomach, I suggest that you avoid surgical videos—this is a time to build confidence, not add discomfort or anxiety.

Educational Resources

- www.niams.nih.gov/Health_Info/Hip_Replacement
- www.mayoclinic.org/tests-procedures/hip-replacement-surgery/basics/definition/prc-20019151
- www.stryker.com/en-us/patients/index.htm
- www.hipsforyou.com
- www.helenhayeshospital.org/total-hip-replacement-surgery-anterior-vs-posterior-approach

PHYSICIAN ASSISTANT

This professional will work beside your surgeon and more than likely apply the staples and/or stitches at the end of your procedure. The physician assistant is often the person who conducts your post-op visits in the weeks, months, and years ahead. Ask about their career and past experience. Understand their methods and how many operations they have assisted your surgeon with, and ask them to describe procedures and tasks they are in charge of during surgery and post-op.

ANESTHESIOLOGIST

This is someone you may not meet until the day of the surgery. Depending on your surgeon, the hospital, and insurance company, the anesthesiologist tends to be a contracted part of the team that is assigned to your surgery by the hospital. If you can find out who you are working with prior to surgery, you can ask about the types of anesthesia that will be used.

In my case, I took additional steps and asked my anesthesiologist if he was willing to repeat positive affirmations to me before, during, and after the surgery. I feel strongly that our subconscious is aware and perceives sounds and words in the operating room. Lucky for me, I was assigned an anesthesiologist who was happy to repeat these affirmations and took my request seriously. If this interests you, a sample list of affirmations is found in Chapter 2.

RADIOLOGIST

I saw my radiologist as a necessary evil. I didn't enjoy standing in awkward positions while being subjected to radiation. These visits left me feeling sore and looking at the X-rays with my doctor were a bit frightening. However, I understood how important these images were to my surgeon. X-rays are maps required to outline a successful outcome. Preparation for a hip replacement requires numerous X-rays. Your surgeon may or may not offer X-ray services on site.

In order for the technician to examine the head of the femur and portions of the pelvis, there are a number of poses you'll be asked to stand or lie in while being X-rayed. For example, posing in a wide stance, pointing your knee away from your body. Sensations range from a bit uncomfortable to fairly painful. I took anti-inflammatories before the appointments and used topical analgesic creams to relieve any achiness.

The X-ray technician will help position you and assist you through the experience. Bring slip-on shorts to wear while X-rayed—shorts that have no metal catches, buttons, or zipper. If you have a thyroid condition, ask for a thyroid guard before being X-rayed to protect you against the excess radiation exposure. I have Hashimoto's disease and always use this guard, even at the dentist's office.

NURSING TEAM

In the surgeon's office, nurses or medical assistants take your vital signs, weigh you, and handle blood draws. Both in and outside the surgery room, the nurses at the hospital will meet you the day of surgery. I suggest introducing yourself, shaking hands, and thanking them in advance for their care. A positive, grateful attitude goes a long way to let these individuals know that you appreciate their hard work, professionalism, and training.

After surgery, these men and women help you with a sponge bath, assist with daily hygiene, help you to and from the bathroom, and manage the tubes/catheters/drains and other devices that will be attached to you. This aspect of caretaking can be embarrassing—I felt much more at ease being on a first-name basis, being able to crack a joke, and using chitchat to distract myself from those uncomfortable yet necessary nursing tasks. There are caretaking moments, especially in the hospital, which breach personal boundaries. Employ humor if it helps and know that you are working with trained professionals. Always speak up if you feel uncomfortable.

PHYSICAL THERAPIST

After surgery, you're taught how to move and how not to move the new joint. The physical therapist is your resident expert and helps you execute these movements perfectly. You will practice walking as soon as possible. This is important, and yes, it will be difficult and painful. Your health and healing depends upon moving. Some patients may attend physical therapy the same day they have surgery. This therapy is the beginning of your rehabilitation. Most patients are offered group-based sessions in a large classroom rather than individual therapy. As you ease into movement and are taught how to safely maneuver, you'll use props such as stairways, bath tubs, and seats of cars. The exercises are a variety of leg lifts and swings that decrease the swelling, increase strength, and help you heal. The therapist might advise a family member or caregiver to attend your physical therapy sessions to better understand how you should move. You may be given an exercise log and guidebook demonstrating your new workout routine. If not, ask for one.

HOME HEALTH AIDE

Depending on your insurance company and directives from your surgeon, you may qualify for home visits from a health professional. This person may be a nurse, medical assistant, or physical therapist. They will assess your progress, see that you are performing your exercises, change bandages, and assess your home environment for safety. I had semiweekly visits for a few weeks and appreciated having a medical professional in my home.

FAMILY MEMBERS AND CAREGIVERS

Many people are able to care for themselves on their own after being discharged from the hospital. Others may feel more comfortable transitioning to a rehabilitation facility. You and your surgeon will decide what is best for you. A family member or caretaker at home with you during the first week or two after surgery can help. They can motivate you to complete daily exercises and assist you with meal preparation, bathing, and dressing. If you do not have anyone to assist you, inform your physical therapist and nursing staff. Your surgeon should be aware of how you will be cared for at home. Inform your doctor if your home has barriers to recovery such as steep stairways. Hospital staff and your surgeon will ensure that you are prepared to go home and live solo if that is your only option. I had minimal help and felt okay on my own after a short time.

CONSIDER THIS

Healing from a joint replacement surgery takes time and effort. Preparing your home and modifying your environment ahead of time will make all the difference toward a more successful and safer recovery. This topic is discussed in detail in Chapter 2.

Patience is crucial during recovery, patience from you and anyone else assisting you. Hip replacement is a major surgery. The procedure nearly removes your leg, removes bone, and replaces the head of the femur with new, artificial parts. Muscle groups are cut and drainage tubes may be placed near the incision site. It's not a pretty picture. There is a great deal of discomfort, swelling, bruising, and pain. This information isn't meant to scare you; only to convey the realities of the experience. Have courage. You can get through this, you will heal, and you'll return to a new quality of life.

Build a relationship with your medical caregivers. Honest and open conversations help you know what to expect. Take a notebook to your doctor visits and write down any questions you may have. Remember that no question is a dumb question.

---

[2] Marchione M. Study: 2 percent of Americans have artificial hips, knees. New Jersey Herald website. Published March 12, 2014. Updated March 26, 2014. Accessed February 17, 2017.

CHAPTER 2
PREPARING FOR SURGERY

*It's better to look ahead and prepare, than to look back
and regret.*
—Jackie Joyner-Kersee

Timing is one benefit of hip replacement surgery. The majority of the procedures are planned well in advance. This timing allows patients to prepare their home, coordinate time off work, and schedule caretaking needs. Added time is also helpful to prepare yourself mentally and emotionally.

There are exceptions to the rule and emergencies occur. A fall or fracture may lead to immediate hip replacement surgery. In those situations, preparation takes place alongside surgery. Whatever your case may be, utilize any time you have to make changes, even if you are coordinating them from your hospital bed. Recruit help if you can.

Begin by taking a thorough look at your home. Modifying common living spaces such as the bedroom, bathroom, and kitchen, sets the stage for a safe recovery. Scan areas for fall hazards, clutter, or narrow walkways. Focus on changes that will help you to maneuver easily while on crutches or using a walker. Many of the changes you make at home may become permanent—enabling you to live safely, effectively, and comfortably. Preventing falls now and in the future is very important. Receiving a hip replacement is a lifestyle change for you and everyone else who lives with you. Whether you have days or weeks to prepare, there are a number of tasks you can address now.

WEEKS PRIOR TO SURGERY

Before buying any medical equipment, review your health plan. If you have a flexible spending account or health savings account, you can use that money to help you pay for home health equipment. Ask friends or family if they have any equipment you can borrow as you recover.

Crutches and dressing tools are provided by the hospital. Beyond that, you'll need a bath chair, a cane, and a raised toilet seat for at least one bathroom. Grab bars for the tub or shower will be helpful too. For moving around, a walker or wheelchair may be useful. I found that having a wheelchair was especially helpful during activities where walking for long periods would be too taxing and tire me out. For example, after my revision surgery I had been on crutches for weeks and my partner took me to the zoo. The sunshine, distraction, and activity boosted my mood, though maneuvering the zoo on crutches would have been exhausting and dangerous for me. A wheelchair helped out immensely. These items can be purchased or even rented at a medical supply outlet, online, or at a local retailer in the pharmacy department.

After surgery, your feet may be swollen and wider than normal for a week or two. A pair of comfortable, sturdy shoes is helpful for the trip home from the hospital and to wear at home while you participate in your physical therapy exercises. Avoid wearing house slippers that are slip-on. Slippers should be shoe-like, wrap around your heel, and have a solid tread. Also, if you have shoes with heels higher than half an inch, it's time to consider getting rid of them. That includes dress shoes, cowboy boots, motorcycle boots, etc. High-heeled shoes are detrimental to the health of your new joint and aren't safe. Wearing heels can cause you to slip and fall, plus they place your hips and spine out of alignment, creating an imbalance. I tossed out dozens of beautiful shoes and boots, begrudgingly resigning myself to the world of flats. Vanity has sometimes led me to test this theory, though my hips and lower back scold me every time I attempt wearing heels that are too high.

Outside of your closet, plan to rearrange anything you use often by placing it at or above hip level. You won't be bending very well for quite some time and bending past 90 degrees is off limits, especially for those receiving a posterior placement. Rearrange cooking tools in your kitchen and personal items in the bathroom and bedroom. Small details like these can help you remain independent and safe during your recovery. Consider the word "safe" your new mantra.

PREPARE A LIVING WILL

This suggestion may seem a bit ominous, but it's not. A living will is simply an investment that protects your wishes and provides you and your family with security. These are health directives that give you control over medical procedures in case of illness. You state what you do and do not wish to happen in certain medical situations. This document will speak for you in case you cannot. Living will forms are specific to the state you live in and are easy to prepare. Provide the hospital and your surgeon with a copy. You can find an advance directives/living will for any state at www.caringinfo.org/i4a/pages/index.cfm?pageid=3289.

VISIT YOUR DENTIST

Dental work may not be very high on your priority list right now, *though it should be.* After hip replacement surgery, recipients are at a higher risk of infection. When I received my first hip replacement in 2011, I was informed that any future medical procedure, including minor or major dental work, would require premedication. Infections can lead to a failed joint and further surgery, even years after a hip replacement. One of my dear friends had a hip replacement after a lifelong career of ballet. She experienced a serious bacterial infection eight years after her hip replacement. This infection invaded the bone surrounding her artificial joint and caused joint failure. In order to treat the infection, a revision surgery was necessary to repair the joint. **If you have time, schedule a dental visit prior to surgery** for a cleaning and complete any necessary dental work as a preventive measure.

In 2015 I visited my dentist to repair a chipped crown and mentioned that I was writing this book. He told me of a recent dental conference he attended where patient premedication was discussed. Treating patients with antibiotics before dental work or other procedures had been considered preventive care and preferred for those who have artificial joints. This recommendation has changed. According to the American Dental Association, as of January 2015, "For patients with prosthetic joint implants, ... antibiotics are not recommended prior to dental procedures to prevent prosthetic joint infections." For any patients who had a history of complications, antibiotics should only be considered after a consultation with the patient and the orthopedic surgeon.[3] This ruling was of great interest to my dentist who had his own reservations regarding excess use of antibiotics. My dentist and many of his colleagues agreed that this cautious approach was a positive change.

The clinical reasoning behind this recommendation is evidence that dental infections are not associated with prosthetic joint infections and antibiotics provided before oral care did not prevent joint implant infections. Situations vary by patient, and if the surgeon deemed that antibiotics would support the health of the patient, the

ADA suggests following medication guidelines. Speak candidly to your dentist about your joint replacement and be aware of these premedication changes. Discuss concerns and know your risk for infection. You, your dentist, and your surgeon can determine if premedication is best for you in the years to come.

MANAGE STRESS

The negative health effects of stress have been researched and well documented. Hip replacement surgery is a strenuous and stressful ordeal. Excess stress can raise blood pressure, decrease immune function, lead to depression, and contribute to sleep problems. Whether you find stress relief with laughter, reading a good book, taking a long bath, or listening to music, find and practice ongoing stress management to aid your recovery and better manage your health. Here are some additional methods to help you de-stress:

- Complementary and alternative therapies such as massage, meditation, and acupuncture top my list for managing stress. Touch is a powerful tool.
- Reiki is a Japanese word meaning universal life energy. This gentle, non-intrusive method can alleviate pain and stress. Reiki practitioners use little to no pressure and follow a series of hand positions on or slightly above the head, shoulders, back, chest, stomach, and limbs. This technique is adaptable to nearly any setting such as hospital bed or chair, and through bandages.
- Distract yourself with good company. Even those who treasure solitude may feel overwhelmed if there is too much alone time throughout recovery. Companionship provides solace and comfort.
- YouTube browsing led me to the videos of Brad Yates and EFT, or Emotional Freedom Technique. Better known as "tapping," this method is designed to gain relief from negative emotion,

stress, and trauma. Find Brad's videos and learn more about EFT at www.bradyates.net.

- Have a pet? Animal therapy does wonders for blood pressure and brings a smile to your face.
- Palming is a simple technique that eases eye strain, moistens dry eyes, and helps you to relax. You can learn more at www.wikihow.com/Do-Palming-Properly.

For those who enjoy a more passive approach toward stress management, I recommend guided imagery. I discovered this audio technique while studying massage therapy. If you aren't familiar with guided imagery, think of it as a scripted daydream designed to promote health and healing. The guided imagery professional I am most familiar with is Belleruth Naparstek, ACSW, BCD, founder of Health Journeys. I wholeheartedly recommend her work. Belleruth's *Stress Management* and *Weight Loss* CDs were already incorporated into my monthly wellness routine. After learning I needed a hip replacement, I purchased another of her titles, *Successful Surgery*. I listened to this CD once or twice a day for weeks prior to my surgery. Gaining my surgeon's permission, I also listened to this audio during my surgery using an MP3 player and earbuds. After surgery, I continued to listen daily while napping for an additional three weeks. You can multitask using guided imagery and listen while you sleep, though don't listen while you operate machinery or drive. This is relaxation time. The audio is just as effective whether you are awake or asleep. The carefully chosen words, well-designed music, and positive affirmations are soothing, supportive, and calming. If you're interested in this method, visit www.healthjourneys.com to learn more about guided imagery.

REMAIN ACTIVE

Yes you have limitations, yes you are in pain and uncomfortable, and yes activity may seem counterintuitive for a person facing hip replacement surgery. HOWEVER, by choosing to exercise in whatever form that you are able, you tap into tremendous benefits physically, emotionally, and mentally. There are a number of activities to participate in even if you are very limited or are seated most of the time. Remember that even moderate to mild activity helps to manage stress, improves your cardiovascular health, and heightens immune function. Even minimal effort will increase your upper body strength and support your heart. Speak to your surgeon or physical therapist for a list of exercises that you can safely participate in before surgery. You are encouraged to exercise daily in the hospital, so buck up and get moving. Your improved health depends on it.

Consider incorporating a method from the list below to keep movement in your day:

- Seated yoga or Tai Chi
- Upper body strength training
- Deep breathing exercises
- Isometric exercises
  - The Royal Canadian Air Force XBX Plan
    www.corvedale.com/5bx/xbxPlan.pdf
  - Sit and Be Fit
    www.sitandbefit.org
- Stretching routines
  - Classical Stretch by Essentrics (Miranda Esmonde-White) www.classicalstretch.com
- Toe-tapping, knee lifts, and ankle rotations

- Find exercise videos on YouTube. Here's an example of cardio activity while seated:
www.youtube.com/watch?v=1CdwOe-5OaA

SUPPLEMENTS AND NUTRITIONAL SUPPORT

Let food be thy medicine, and medicine be thy food.
—Hippocrates

A wholesome healthy meal plan is **powerful**. When you are ill, in pain, swollen, and preparing your body for surgery, your body requires the nutrients, minerals, and calories that whole foods provide. Quality nutrition supports digestive health, helps to minimize inflammation, and fights off infection. If you need support improving your meal plans, speak to a registered dietitian. Resources in this book, including my own website, offer free online support, recipes, and meal plans. Simple and inexpensive foods such as potatoes, brown rice, beans, and yams are nutritional powerhouses and can be prepared quickly. These starchy foods contain nearly all the nutrients needed for good health and are very satisfying.

Supplements such as herbs, homeopathic remedies, and vitamins contribute to improved health and speed the healing process. My doctor provided me with specific guidelines of what I should and should not take prior to surgery. The supplements that helped me were specific to my own conditions and might not be the best for you. That caution being noted, one homeopathic remedy receiving positive attention in the health community is arnica. Arnica is extracted from a flowering plant, and contains properties that heal bruises, decrease swelling, and lessen pain. Arnica tablets can be taken internally and gels or creams are available for topical use.

35

Always seek guidance from a medical professional prior to use. Some people may be allergic to arnica or taking medications that can negatively interact with any homeopathic treatment.

I was introduced to arnica while studying massage therapy. I began using this professionally with massage clients and kept the topical form of arnica in my medicine cabinet. I noticed bruises healed more quickly after applying arnica gel and pain decreased. Both my surgeon and my family practitioner recommended that I begin using arnica tablets immediately after my hip replacement surgery. I began my directed regimen as soon as I regained my appetite and continued taking the tablets until all the staples were removed. After the incision was closed, I switched to the topical gel and applied it around the incision site to minimize swelling and bruising.

For more information about arnica, visit:

- www.umm.edu/health/medical/altmed/herb/Arnica
- www.boironusa.com/?products=/Arnica30c-pellets

Remember to speak to your doctor before using arnica in any form.

Another homeopathic remedy I began the day of surgery were Hyland's Bioplasma cell salts. These cell salts are small tablets that melt under the tongue and are made up of, you guessed it, salt. According to the Hyland website, "Cell Salts stimulate the body's natural healing mechanisms to satisfy mineral imbalances." They are based on specific minerals to support the body while healing. My family practitioner recommended that I take these for 60 days after my surgery. You can read more about cell salts at www.hylands.com/media/news/history-cell-salts.

WEEK OF SURGERY

HOME PREPARATION

Bathroom

It's time to incorporate the home health devices I mentioned earlier, if you haven't already. Install a raised toilet seat in the bathroom you use most often. You'll find bathroom visits a bit more comfortable using this seat riser for a number of weeks after surgery. The raised seat eases the effort it takes bending toward the toilet. Raised toilet seats are affordable, can be purchased online, and insurance or flexible spending/HSA dollars may help defer the cost.

A bath chair is a must since a full shower or bath won't be an option until the incision is fully healed and the staples or stitches are removed. A bath chair is essentially a small plastic seat with drainage holes, metal legs, and rubber feet for stability. Bath chairs are designed to fit comfortably in a standard tub, are simple to clean, lightweight, and easy to store. Some bath chairs are a basic bench style. Others provide a back rest or even add arm support to help you lift yourself from a seated position. Metal safety bars in the tub, shower, and next to the toilet add safety and stability. If your bathroom does not have these fixtures in place, they can be installed easily. Safety bars for the shower or tub are available in models using strong suction cups if you are opposed to attaching a permanent fixture. Remove all bath rugs and loose items on the floor or bathroom walkway that can cause you to slip and fall. Make sure there is a place near the tub and toilet to rest your crutches or cane so they do not fall away from you. Sometimes you may sit down and find that your walking supports have gotten away from you and you may need to call for help!

Bathroom preparation also depends on what type of hip replacement you are receiving, your current health, and how active you are. If you receive a posterior hip replacement, the incision is deeper and requires a longer recovery time. You may receive interior stitching with an anterior hip replacement; meaning you might be able to get the incision wet earlier than a posterior recipient can (you should receive clear instructions from your hospital staff or surgeon regarding bathing before leaving the hospital). Additional bathing aids you might feel useful:

- Long-handled brush to clean your back and legs; remember that bending will be uncomfortable, and discouraged
- Foot brush or foot scrubber (pads that attach to the tub floor)
- Bath seat cushion
- Large cup or pitcher for rinsing
- Handheld shower head
- Rubber safety mat
- Emergency whistle (most people prefer to bathe and handle hygiene alone, a whistle nearby is a great alert in case of a fall or slip)

Bedroom

Purchase extra pillows for comfort and to support you during the recovery period and beyond. The ideal sleep position for six weeks up to six months is on your back with pillow support between the knees and feet. Side lying, especially for posterior placement, can place you at a higher risk for dislocation until the muscle and bone have had time to mend. Positioning a pillow between your knees will keep your hips apart and prevent you from crossing your leg during sleep. These supports help you avoid dislocation. During my hospital stay, the nurses positioned a wedge-shaped pillow between my legs to keep me from moving around too much, though this restriction also led to lower back pain and stiffness. I'll be honest; my first month at home I found that getting to sleep and staying asleep was challenging. Most nights I was uncomfortable and received most of my rest in batches and constant napping. Pain medication helped me fall asleep, though I never slept soundly. My partner and I shared a large king-sized bed yet my needs were disruptive and his sleep suffered as well. Be aware of the needs of both people if you share a bed. There may be a period of time where sleeping separate is more comfortable. We were limited to one bed and dealt with the temporary lack of sleep.

A unique aspect of my bed is that it was built with a wood base set fairly high from the ground. This extra height from the floor was helpful because lowering myself into a bed of more normal height may have been awkward and painful. When you get into bed, you will face away from the mattress, back up against the bed, and sit down. Once you are seated fully and have rested your crutches or cane nearby, shift your hips further onto the mattress, using your arms and upper body to support you. When you feel stable, turn your torso and hips to raise your legs onto your bed. This motion will take practice and feel incredibly awkward. You may have to lean back and even inch yourself across the mattress to pull your legs up off the floor. Do not do this alone until you are confident that you have the strength and mobility to position yourself safely. A few added steps are required when you are unable to bend and twist. This applies to all furniture and bathroom fixtures in the house as you recover and get accustomed to moving safely with your new joint. Lowering and raising yourself from the bed, chairs, a car, and couches may be challenging. You will rely on your upper body strength. Again, be sure to remove throw rugs and tuck away any cords or obstacles on the floor and walkway that could cause you to slip and fall. Falling can lead to dislocation and more surgery.

Kitchen

Make note of any foods, dishes, pans, or culinary gadgets that are used often in your kitchen. These items, and anything you need for cooking and cleaning, should be placed *at or above hip level*. Rearrange items in your refrigerator as well—after coming home from the hospital, you will be sore, stiff, and unable to bend. Save room in your freezer for ice packs—the hospital should send some home with you to treat the inflammation. You'll find that using ice afterward can decrease swelling and minimize pain.

Portion-sized meals such as soups, casseroles, stews, and convenience foods such as oatmeal packets, frozen vegetables, waffles, precooked rice, and baked potatoes are comfort foods that are nourishing, simple to prepare, and easy to digest. Recovery from this surgery requires a lot of rest, so keep your meals simple and easy.

Try to get assistance at least during the first week or two. Perhaps family members or neighbors can prepare meals for you. For those who will be making their own meals, take advantage of convenience appliances such as the microwave, slow cooker, rice cooker, toaster, and blender. If you are able, prepare and freeze simple meals prior to surgery. This can save time, energy, and money.

Living Room

For comfort and ease of movement, rearrange furniture and widen walkways to help you move with any assistive devices such as your crutches or cane. If you have a coffee table or tight quarters, measure the area to see how well you will be able to move around after you come home from the hospital. Lowering yourself to a standard couch may be a bit awkward during the first few weeks, especially if you will be on your own. A recliner can feel comfortable, especially if you have foot support and are able to raise your legs. Sitting for long periods slows circulation; it's best to keep your feet elevated. While you rest, toe-tapping and ankle pump exercises promote circulation. An extra pillow or two to support your back and legs plus a blanket nearby help you remain comfortable. Before lowering yourself to any piece of furniture, be sure you can get back up again. Chairs with both back and armrests provide better support though aren't always the most comfortable. You may find that you spend most of your time resting in bed and will use up a lot of energy taking yourself to and from the bathroom and completing your daily exercises.

PERSONAL ITEMS

I've mentioned swelling, and will repeat it here. Do not underestimate how much your body is going to change. A large incision and a long piece of titanium are going to be inserted from your hip socket midway into the length of your femur, which means a lot of post-operative inflammation. Plus, the incision is covered with thick bandages. Your hip will feel and look misshapen, as though you've got a literal one-sided "bubble butt." Since you'll have a bit more padding to cover, you may need to go shopping for a few personal items.

Clothing

Once you are home, wear clothing that is simple and easy for you to move in, use the bathroom, bathe, and change bandages. Nothing in your closet is going to fit well until the swelling goes down. If you don't own a pair already, purchase some elastic waist pajama pants that are easy to slide on and off over the bandages and compression stockings. Oversized fleece, satin, or cotton pajama pants are options that work well and are comfortable. Avoid robes with long cords or waist belts, this type of clothing is cumbersome and can tangle around your feet and crutches. Find items that you can walk in that won't cause you to trip.

To dress yourself, the physical therapist will teach you to use dressing tools and "grabber sticks" to lift pant legs and help you maneuver clothing. The dressing tools are a bit awkward, take a deep breath ... you'll get the hang of it. At least they are durable for times when you throw them against the wall in frustration. Understand that the time it takes to return to your pre-surgery shape is different for everyone. When I returned to work after two weeks, I found that I had no slacks that would fit comfortably over the bandaging. It took about six weeks after my first hip replacement for the swelling to subside so I could fit more comfortably in my normal clothing. Due to the sensitivity of the muscles and scar, I preferred wearing looser clothing for the first three months, especially at work.

Compression Hose

After surgery, you will wear the thigh-high compression hose that I mentioned earlier. These are very tight stockings and are tough to put on. They are also hideous and uncomfortable. However, compression hose are also *crucial* for your recovery since they promote circulation throughout the entire leg. Compression stockings are worn day and night on both legs for at least six weeks after surgery. During surgery, major arteries and blood vessels are cut. While they heal, the compression hose will stabilize blood pressure, can prevent blood clots or deep vein thrombosis, decrease the achy and heavy feeling in your legs, and help to prevent varicose veins. There is an art to putting on compression hose. The nursing staff and physical therapist will help you and provide you with a special dressing tool. Putting a small amount of cornstarch or baby powder on your legs can help the hose slide on easier. Also, wearing rubber gloves provides you with a better grip when you are pulling the stockings on. Obtain at least two pairs of compression stockings so you can alternate on laundry day. The pair you receive in the hospital are white. If you want darker colors for work outfits, they can be purchased online or at a medical supply outlet. Flexible spending plans/HSA dollars may also help with the cost. Wear them as directed.

Underwear

Whatever size you currently wear, purchase a few pairs at least one or two sizes larger to accommodate the swelling of your hip until your incision heals and the inflammation goes down. Women may want to opt for the larger full-sized panty or a short boxer. Men may also want to opt for a roomy boxer. An extra stretchy waist band will feel more comfortable over the bandages and help for the extra time you'll need getting to and from the bathroom. Plan ahead or risk a possibly embarrassing plea for help.

Toenails

This may seem silly to mention, but remember to take care of your toenails *before* your surgery. Bending toward your feet comfortably isn't going to be happening on your own for several weeks. Considering small details like these help put into perspective how much your life is going to change during recovery. In the months to follow, invest in a pedicure; it is worth the money for women and men to let the nail pro save you from bending forward! Plus, pedicures feel delightful.

Hair

Take long showers before your surgery—trust me, you are going to miss the sensation of standing in your shower or soaking in the bath for a while. You won't be able to wash your own hair for a few weeks after surgery. For a posterior hip replacement, you may be able to shower after four to five weeks, anterior placement may allow you to shower after two or three weeks. Consider scheduling a weekly wash and style at your hairdresser or barber for the first three weeks. If a hair stylist doesn't fit your budget, simply purchase dry shampoo and opt for a low-maintenance hairstyle.

Medications, Vitamins, and Supplements

Your doctor and hospital staff will advise you on what medicines and vitamins you should and shouldn't be taking during the weeks and days prior to surgery. This also includes any topical creams, herbal remedies, homeopathic medicines, sublingual dissolving tablets, patches, or inhalants. Inform your medical team of anything you are using, whether it is prescription, over the counter, or recreational, including stimulants such as tobacco or synthetic nicotine. The hospital I worked with also provided a check-in call the day before surgery. This call was conducted by a registered nurse who discussed my medications and was available for any questions or concerns regarding my stay. If in doubt, speak to your doctor or pharmacist.

Help from Family or Others

Hopefully, you have someone in your world that will drive you to the hospital and stay with you the day of surgery. If not, speak to the hospital staff and notify them if you are going to arrive on your own. Many hospitals have patient advocates and caring nursing staff that can spend extra time chatting with you and provide a hand to hold if you feel frightened. You will need someone to drive you home. Even if you go directly home rather than a rehabilitation facility, it's a good idea to have someone check in on you or spend at least some time with you during the first week or two. I was lucky that my father was retired and able to visit me every day after I returned home from the hospital. This isn't mandatory of course. Many people return home after receiving a hip replacement and are fully capable of caring for their needs. I found my father's company to be reassuring and comforting since my biggest fear was losing my balance and falling. Bottom line is to decide what feels best for you, what you are able to afford, and take advantage of any assistance you can.

I was honestly much more self-sufficient than I had imagined. My dad is entertaining though a bit old school. I was preparing his meal and mine plus being my own cheerleader during my exercises, so after a week I sent him back home. If you do have help it's a good idea to chat about expectations and tell them what you need and expect. People really do appreciate direction and want to know how they can help. I'm an awesome cook and my dad knew I wouldn't want anything he would make, so his presence was the perfect help for me.

DAY BEFORE SURGERY

This is an important day. Recruit help and look through your home to see if you've missed any preparations or need to finish some final rearranging. Enjoy quality meals today to fill your body with nutrients—add extra fiber in the form of vegetables, fruits, and plenty of whole grains. These foods will help you avoid the post-op constipation following anesthesia and pain medications. You will fast from food and beverages this evening. Stay hydrated and rinse your mouth if it feels dry throughout the night. Do not swallow any fluids; an empty stomach is required the day of surgery.

Pack for your hospital stay accordingly, expecting to be there at least two or more nights—your doctor or hospital staff may provide a list giving you an idea of what you will need. You should receive a surgical prep kit for your shower or bath the day of surgery—this includes a special soap to be used at the surgical site. Make sure after you bathe that you do not use lotion, perfumes, or creams. If you shave, this is a good day to take care of that final hygiene item so you won't be bothered with that task in the weeks to follow. If you like the idea of not needing to shave, then by all means enjoy that furry feeling. Men with hair on their legs and hips may be asked to shave, though most hospitals prefer to handle that task the day of surgery. Select a comfortable outfit to wear to the hospital. Remember to bring oversized bottoms and flat shoes for your ride home.

Leave valuables and personal items such as your cell phone, jewelry, wallet, identification, glasses, and hygiene items with family and friends. Anything else you truly need can be brought to you after you are settled in your hospital room. Besides my clothing and essentials, I brought along the following:

- MP3 player and earbuds
- Arnica and other homeopathic remedies
- Hand sanitizer
- Lip balm
- Lemon essential oil and cotton balls

Why lemon essential oil? Lemon has antibacterial and antiviral properties ... plus I enjoy the uplifting smell. I placed a few drops on a cotton ball and swabbed my food tray, wiped down the hospital bed rails, cleaned off the television remote control, and placed a scented cotton ball in my pillowcase. Hospitals have a medicinal smell; adding the refreshing scent of lemon to my pillow helped me sleep and boosted my spirits.

Your shower or bath at home today will be one of the final full soaks you'll experience until your incision heals; enjoy it and hopefully you rest well and sleep soundly tonight. Luxuriate and soak in the tub if you are able. Tomorrow is a big day!

DAY OF SURGERY

Do not forget that you are fasting. No food, no beverages, no mints, not even a stick of gum. Ideally you are scheduled for an early-morning surgery and won't have too much time on your hands. If you experience dry mouth, simply rinse your mouth with water and spit it out.

The morning of my first hip replacement surgery, my significant other and I went to the gym for a full upper body weight training workout. Is this suggestion an option for you? That depends on you and your activity level. The morning of my second hip replacement surgery, I still exercised to a certain degree. By my third revision surgery, even though I was on crutches I still went to the gym for an upper body routine that morning. For me, exercise is therapeutic for my body, mind, and emotional well-being. Getting out of the house, distracting my mind, and focusing on what I was able to do rather than worrying about the surgery was a boost for my self-confidence. Exercise provides energy, promotes circulation, and enhances your immune function. I viewed my time at the gym those days as added insurance to protect me against infection, assuring me that I was going to be okay. Surgery is scary. Invest a bit of time this morning in an activity that brings you joy and peace of mind. That activity might not be exercise—perhaps listen to a beautiful piece of music, watch a short comedy, meditate, or watch the sunrise. You're going to be okay!

Final to-dos this morning before you head to the hospital:

- **Tidy up.** During your preoperative shower this morning, you'll use medicated soap to minimize bacteria on your skin. This decreases your risk for infection. Follow the directions carefully and take this task seriously. Remember, do not apply lotions, creams, or scent to your skin—specifically at the surgery site. Keep your skin clean and dry before you dress.

- **Check your suitcase** one more time in case there are any items you need or should leave behind. Pajamas...yes, money...won't need it, this book...yes, teddy bear and a deck of cards...why not!

- **Maintain a positive attitude!** I kept the radio on my favorite radio station, KRCL 90.9. This is a community-based station in Salt Lake City. Listen to soothing music, say a prayer, or listen to guided imagery to relieve any anxiety or preoperative jitters. I spent a few minutes to meditate, and sought humor throughout the morning—even nervous laughter is laughter!

When you arrive at the hospital and are taken to the preparation room, you'll be asked to put on a hospital gown and a full leg compression stocking on the nonsurgical leg—the other stocking will be placed on you after surgery. These are the compression hose I described earlier under personal items. As much as they are uncomfortable and incredibly difficult to put on, the support they provide for circulation and healing is necessary and a significant factor in how well you heal. After surgery, you may want to stop wearing them sooner than you should. You'll find that you actually feel better when you are wearing your compression hose. I experienced this a few weeks after my first surgery. After removing a pair on wash day, I felt my legs deserved a break and needed to "air out" before hoisting on a clean pair. It didn't take long before I felt shaky in my movements and a bit light-headed. That was strong feedback for me and I wore my hose religiously from that point forward.

The last item you'll put on to prepare for surgery is a hairnet. However your hair looks prior to surgery, expect it to look like hell for at least the next three to four days, mine sure did! I love my hair and it really bothered me wearing the hairnet. Isn't it silly what goes through your mind and what becomes a priority in times of stress and drastic change? Thinking back, I'm glad I had this added last-minute distraction to take my mind off the surgery. If you have a low-maintenance hairstyle, then you're a lucky duck!

The waiting game prior to surgery is different for everyone—there are always other patients scheduled before and after you. A hospital is a busy place so it's best to be prepared for the day to run late. Ideally, everything will run on schedule, and you'll be whisked away and promptly put to "sleep" as your star medical team takes good care of you. If you have a family member or friend with you, enjoy their company and chat, flip through a magazine, and if you feel frightened or emotional, let it out. It's okay to ask for a hug or hold someone's hand (even if that means asking a nurse). It's natural and understandable to ask for a box of tissues and cry. This is a *major surgery* you are embarking upon. Deep breathing exercises are a great source of comfort and can calm your nerves.

Once it's time for you to move toward the surgery room, those accompanying you are generally directed to a waiting room or cafeteria. Now it's just you and the hospital staff wheeling your bed down the corridors. My family said they were treated like gold and given snacks and beverages while they waited for my surgery updates. But don't quote me on this, every hospital is different. The moment I headed to the surgery room is when I felt as though I entered a television drama watching the ceiling lights pass by above me. Aside from the funky visuals, my earbuds provided the contrast of relaxing melodies and comforting words to help me take in this surreal view. Hospitals just weren't places I was incredibly familiar with.

I had been fortunate to avoid patient status at a hospital since 1987 when I gave birth to my one and only son ... so this experience was completely foreign to me. When you arrive outside the surgery room, you may be tucked to one side in the corridor. This was unnerving for me; I didn't really care for extra time to view these sterile surroundings with all sorts of surgical equipment in plain sight. So once again I turned inward, focused on the audio and closed my eyes, which helped to tune out the strange sounds of this part of the hospital. Luckily, this time in the hallway was short for me—I soon saw the friendly faces of my surgeon, physician assistant, and anesthesiologist.

I felt lucky to have a medical team that supported my desire to wear earbuds and agreed to talk to me during the surgery, encouraging and reassuring me with positive affirmations. Positive affirmation scripts can be found online or you can simply write a few simple upbeat sentences that have meaning to you. Below I've listed a few of the affirmations I asked to be read while I was unconscious:

"You can be confident in me as your surgeon. I will take good care of you."

"You are safe and in the care of professionals, we are taking good care of you."

"You are breathing slowly and your heartbeat is steady."

"The surgery is going really well. This is a success."

"You are going to recover well."

"Your body is already beginning to heal."

"Your new joint is going to help you live a full life."

"Your bone is accepting the new joint, this is a good fit."

When you are taken into the surgery room and transferred to the surgical table, time passes quickly. You are put to sleep and are in the hands of professionals. Trust that they have your best interest at heart. Have faith in a positive outcome.

Are you ready? Use this checklist to help you prepare for surgery.

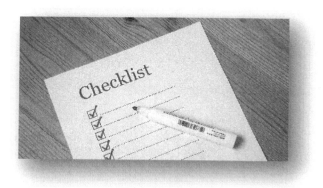

SURGERY PREPARATION CHECKLIST
- ☐ Schedule dental visit before surgery
- ☐ Exercise—safely continue regular physical activity
  - ○ My preoperative routine included upper body resistance training (weights), stretching, and chair aerobics. Check with your doctor for exercises that are best **for you**.
- ☐ Prepare your home
  - ○ Bedroom
  - ○ Bathroom
  - ○ Kitchen
  - ○ Living areas

- o Clothing
- o Nails and hair
- ☐ Meal planning—examples of simple dishes
  - o Potato corn chowder
  - o Chili
  - o Casseroles
  - o Spaghetti
  - o Oatmeal with added fruit, cinnamon, and nuts
  - o Enchiladas
  - o Sandwich fixings
- ☐ Family and caregiver support—who will help you?
- ☐ Prepare a living will—leave a copy with family and provide a copy for the hospital
- ☐ Medication list for the hospital and pharmacist
- ☐ Day of surgery
  - o Stress management
  - o Check hospital bag—do you have everything you need?

---

[3] Sollecito TP, Abt E, Lockhart PB, et al. The use of prophylactic antibiotics prior to dental procedures in patients with prosthetic joints. Journal of the American Dental Association. 2015;146(1): 11–16. Published January 2015. Accessed February 16, 2017.

CHAPTER 3
RECOVERY BEGINS—YOUR HOSPITAL STAY

The reason why not everyone manages to take the healing process as far as it can go is that we differ drastically in our ability to mobilize it.
—Deepak Chopra, M.D. (Journey Into Healing)

The surgery is over, hooray! Healing begins now. Expect to stay in the hospital for at least a few days; your surgeon will discuss this with you, and depending on the rate of your recovery, you may go home early or need to stay a bit longer. I stayed in the hospital for three nights with each of my surgeries.

As the anesthesia clears from your system, the groggy feeling will fade and your head won't feel quite so fuzzy. Your body has been given ample doses of pain medication, and you may feel as though you are a foreigner in your own body. You'll notice a lot of bandaging and ice packs on your hip, perhaps a drainage tube around the incision site, a catheter will have been inserted during surgery, and there will be an IV in your hand or arm. You may be on oxygen for a period of time. Your upper torso will be raised slightly, a wedge-shaped pillow will separate your knees, and your feet will be partially raised. Along your lower body, each leg will be covered with a compression stocking. At your feet, a compression wrap and pump provide intermittent pressure to support circulation.

For those who have experienced surgery and a hospital stay before, this might not seem odd—I felt as though I had landed on the moon. I scanned the entire scene trying to make sense of my surroundings.

I've always thought of a hospital room as gloomy, a bit ominous, a little creepy, and fairly depressing. This isn't necessarily the case since many hospitals are filled with plants, art, colored walls, and music. I asked nursing staff a multitude of questions about each and every device that was attached to me. It was important to me to understand the purpose of each device, tube, and needle. This enabled me to focus on how they were helping me. You and your medical team each have a role to play during this healing process. During this fragile time, the best things we can do for ourselves is to rest, speak up if we're uncomfortable, and make wise choices as our appetite returns.

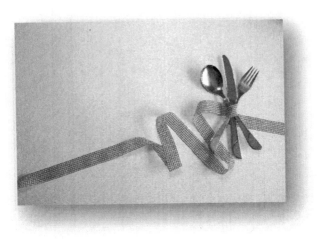

NOURISHMENT

After surgery, most people will regain an appetite quickly and are ready for a meal within an hour or so after waking. You may experience an upset stomach—trust your instincts, you will know if you feel like eating. This is a time when your body is in dire need of nutrients and quality calories. After all, you have survived a lengthy surgery and traumatic procedure. Your taste buds may guide your eyes on the hospital menu ... but use common sense and choose your meals wisely. Hospital menus are designed by registered dietitians and now more than ever you'll discover tasty, appetizing, and beautiful meals to help you get well. Hospital menus offer heart-friendly dishes, vegan options, low-sodium meals, and typically, a calorie count. Do yourself a favor and treat your body to a wholesome feast. Your body is full of anesthesia—the chemicals that were used to put you to sleep during the operation also put your colon to sleep. Eating lots of fiber and foods rich in vitamins will help support powerful detoxifying organs such as your liver and stimulate your intestines. This is my delicate way of saying ... you want to have a bowel movement *on your own* before leaving the hospital. A sleepy colon is not pleasant and after a few days will feel very uncomfortable! If things don't get moving on your own, the nursing staff will be happy to give you an enema. That isn't my idea of a good time. Food is your friend, especially foods high in fiber.

Food, meal plans, and diet are touchy subjects. This is not a diet book. My suggestions are based on personal experience, my educational background, and simply put, what has worked for me. I offer these suggestions as a way to assist you toward a strong recovery and improved health.

A focus on nutrition supports health and healing. Hip replacement recipients are encouraged to maintain a healthy weight. This is, of course, sound advice for everyone. Eating a diet of whole foods helps you stay lean and avoid excess pressure on your new joint. I mentioned this ratio earlier within the Worksheet: Questions for your Surgeon section and emphasize it again. Did you realize that **five pounds of excess body weight places 25 pounds of pressure on a joint**? My surgeon informed me of this, and I stress it here to help you understand how impactful a small amount of weight can be in regards to the health and longevity of your artificial joint. If you have some weight to lose, five pounds will make a tremendous difference.

To keep my own weight within a healthy range, I follow the dietary recommendations from the McDougall Program. The book, *The Starch Solution*, by Dr. John McDougall and the 10-day free program outlined on his website have helped me feel better than ever. The ingredients of his meal plan are simple and affordable—his suggestion is to eat as our ancestors have for thousands of years by eating potatoes, beans, legumes, whole grains, vegetables, and fruits. I've listed some information in the resource section—there are hundreds of delicious and easy recipes online and as I mentioned, a free 10-day program to get you started.

Dr. McDougall and his wife practice what they preach and have maintained great health and lean weight for decades. Check out the website www.drmcdougall.com/health/education/free-mcdougall-program for meal plans, recipes, and free webinars. Nutrition is powerful medicine.

For more information, I recommend:

- *Forks Over Knives*, documentary and cookbook www.forksoverknives.com
- *The Starch Solution*, by Dr. John A. McDougall and Mary McDougall
- *The Healthiest Diet on the Planet*, by Dr. John A. McDougall and Mary McDougall
- *The China Study*, by Dr. T. Colin Campbell and Dr. Thomas M. Campbell II

FEED YOUR MIND

Your brain also enjoys added starches in your diet since starches provide glucose. Our brains use a lot of energy and consume about 20 percent of our daily calories. The fuel of choice for the brain is glucose. Another way to feed your mind during recovery is to manage stress. I lean toward the alternative approaches especially in regards to managing stress and pain. You'll read more about pain management techniques in the next chapter. Alternative options such as guided imagery are low cost or free, with no negative side effects. If you opted for some guided imagery before or even during surgery, continue using the CD or online options to help you relax during your hospital stay. Your family and friends may have brought along your cell phone, laptop, or other devices to keep you company. Use your gadgets to stream music, listen to an audio book, or relax with guided imagery. Try this 15-minute guided imagery technique for free at the following website address: www.healthjourneys.com/Main/FreeGuidedImagery.

PREPARE FOR MOVEMENT

Your energy level will be low but you are still expected to be with the physical therapist either the day of surgery or the day after. These early days of exercise set a strong foundation for the weeks ahead. You'll feel slow, sluggish, awkward, and uncomfortable. You're asking your body to move with new equipment—be patient and maintain a slow, steady pace. You'll experience improvements every day.

Movement will help you heal, decrease the inflammation, and encourage new bone growth. Your surgeon and physical therapist will outline specifics for you based on your circumstances; pay attention to the serious restrictions and movement no-no's that are important to adhere to. As you progress from a walker to using crutches or a cane, there are some movements that will require care and consideration. Listen to your body and notice what motions are especially challenging.

PHYSICAL THERAPY

I have three suggestions for you: Pay attention, participate, and work hard! The smallest steps and tiniest movements will leave you feeling as if your butt is full of lead and that you are a toddler learning to walk again. There is an element of truth to these feelings—during hip replacement surgery, a bit of extra weight from your new artificial joint is installed and the physical therapist is teaching you to walk with an internal assistive device. Your physical therapy protocol will vary depending on your age, ability, and whether you received a posterior or anterior placement. Your surgeon, nursing staff, and physical therapist will discuss the movements, exercises, and most importantly provide directions on *what not to do.*

Take advantage of your therapy time; you'll learn how to modify your motions, everyday tasks, and home environment to support you now and in the future. Your pain may cause hesitation and a tendency to avoid movement. Find a way to stay motivated. Your recovery period is a time to move and exercise. Simply be cautious and consistent with your new fitness routine.

A small walk down the hospital corridor the day of surgery is standard after a hip replacement. I was amazed at how difficult it was to walk. I felt determined and challenged myself to go a little further every walk that followed. Nurses and physical therapists will encourage and stay near you, though your own self-determination is the driving force to speed your recovery. Initially, I used a walker for the first bionic stroll since I was attached to quite a few hoses and tubes. During physical therapy, you may or may not progress to using crutches. I was able to make that transition and elected for shorter crutches rather than the traditional taller crutches that rest under the armpit. You'll find that you rely much more on your upper body strength during recovery. Shoulders and hands will feel sore, and you may build up a callous or two. Stretch your arms, shoulders, neck, and hands to reduce any tension.

People closest to you may be interested in understanding the mechanics of this new joint. Ask if they can attend physical therapy with you. Having others at home who know your limitations and restrictions can encourage your recovery and be supportive as activities are modified. These replacement parts do enable us to move more freely once we are fully recovered. That is the miracle of this surgery—a level of freedom and independence is restored.

BATHING

Oh the joyous experience of hospital stays—the thin billowy backless gown, tousled hair, using a bedpan, being poked and prodded throughout the night for blood draws, noisy corridors 24/7, and sponge baths. Having a nurse assist me with bathing was very uncomfortable—"suck it up and get it over with" was the thought running through my mind. I didn't like the smell of my room let alone the smell of myself, so I knew a bath was definitely needed. Thankfully, nurses are experts at helping you wash—they're very discreet and speed through this task. Once the catheter is removed and you are making your way to the restroom on your own; washing your face and brushing your teeth can feel like quite the accomplishment.

If you were living independently and taking care of yourself prior to surgery you may find it frustrating to have simple freedoms such as bathroom tasks taken away from you. Handling your bathroom routine, even if it is just brushing your teeth, is a task to master quickly. This skill goes beyond taking care of our bodily functions. If you consider the typical layout of a hospital room, the pathway to the restroom isn't always nearest the bed. In addition, there are barriers that may cause a fall such as medical equipment in the room, heavy doors, and devices attached to you. Pain medication dulls our senses and reflexes as well; your body won't respond as quickly as your mind believes it can. An everyday journey is now complex though it also teaches you to maneuver and regain balance. You'll require help initially. Nursing staff will monitor your progress and help you along as needed.

Just a reminder. This book is based around my personal experience; your situation may be similar, or it may be dramatically different. Even with the same type of surgery, we all are going to heal a bit differently and will have unique experiences with the outcome. Bathing is no different—some surgeons may give you a more lenient timeline on when you can shower and expose the incision to water. The main reason to wait is to **avoid infection**. Any infection to incisions this deep in the body can be deadly. Follow your doctor's orders. My surgeon preferred that I wait until after the staples and stitches were removed and the incision fully closed before I was able to shower—for me that meant about four weeks. That was a LONG, LONG time for me to use a bath chair in a standard tub and basically clean myself using washcloths, cups, and buckets. To make this awkward way of bathing less uncomfortable, I would increase the heat in the bathroom so I wouldn't catch a chill and make sure everything I needed was ready before undressing. Revisit the section on home preparation and how to best modify your own bathroom to support you during recovery.

In regards to washing your hair, unless you have a sink and someone to help you, this can be a problem. As I mentioned in an earlier chapter, consider taking advantage of a hairdresser nearby to wash and dry your hair at least for the first couple of weeks. Call ahead to ensure that the salon or barber staff can accommodate a person post-op who is on crutches or a walker. Ideally their hair washing stations will have chairs with wide seats and enable you to raise your feet. Leaning back without having your feet raised can put a strain on your lower back and hips. Pressure on the bandaged area in a snug chair can be harmful. Plus, this semi-reclined position makes it challenging getting *out* of the chair with or without help. I found a salon that was able to assist me and scheduled weekly appointments until I was able to shower on my own. My mother drove me to my appointments until I was able to drive and I enjoyed the extra pampering while someone else cared for my hair, especially during the scalp massage.

LEAVING THE HOSPITAL—REHAB FACILITY OR HOME?

A day or two after your surgery you will have attended a few physical therapy sessions and seen your doctor for some post-op assessments. Many people decide long before surgery whether they feel comfortable going home right away or if transitioning to a rehabilitation facility would be best. This is entirely up to your surgeon and yourself. The discussion of insurance and if you can afford a rehab facility is an important factor. If you have a home with lots of stairs, no one to help you, aren't healing as well as your surgeon would like to see, or would feel more comfortable with added help, then a rehab center might be a good fit.

I knew ahead of time that I lacked the funds and insurance coverage for this option. I returned to home since I lived in an apartment without stairs and had family available to stay with me during the day. Ideally, you will learn how to walk safely on stairs during physical therapy in the hospital, though if you have them at home, a few weeks of avoiding them will keep you safe. When you return to your own bed, you may find that you sleep more soundly simply because you aren't interrupted throughout the night with blood draws and countless hospital staff in and out of the room all hours of the day. On the other hand, if you have pre-existing conditions or had a complicated surgery, sleeping in a facility with around-the-clock care may provide more comfort and security until you are feeling well enough to return home. Consider your options and speak to your surgeon about what is most suitable for you.

Prior to discharge, your physical therapy team will provide you with equipment and tools for use at home—generally they are your crutches, a grabber tool, and a gadget to help you put on your compression stockings. These are billed items; check with your insurance plan to see if they are covered and included with your procedure. The grabbing tool is essential for dressing and handy when you drop items, need to reach a stray sock in the dryer, pick up the newspaper, etc. This grabber helps you avoid bending and is a great tool to keep with you even after you are able to drive and return to work. The discharge nurse may give you a reusable bag that was used for your ice packs. Ask for a few extra to have on hand for rotation. In the weeks to follow, ice will continue to decrease swelling and help with pain. Home care visits are typically discussed prior to surgery and reassessed while you are in the hospital.

Depending on your recovery rate these visits may increase or decrease based on your needs and insurance coverage. I had home care visits twice a week for the first two weeks for bandage changes and exercise assistance. Afterward, my partner changed the dressings for me.

THE RIDE HOME—GETTING INTO YOUR CAR

After receiving your prescriptions, you'll be taken out of the hospital by wheelchair and, hopefully, given added help to get into whatever vehicle that is taking you home. Have a discussion with the family member or friend who is picking you up about getting you in and out of the car. During physical therapy, there is typically a practice vehicle to get in and out of—this teaches you how to move each leg in and out of a vehicle safely. Ask your physical therapy team if your family member can tag along and watch the process so they better understand your limitations. A lower vehicle such as a sedan can be just as challenging as a high-profile vehicle like a truck or van. Either way, do your best and ask that two people are available to help you in and out of the vehicle for this first post-op ride. Your aim is for slow, steady movements.

My significant other owned a Ford Ranger. He adjusted the passenger seat back as far as it could go and lowered the back rest just a bit to widen the entrance to the cab of the truck. It was January in Utah, so it was snowy and cold and I was eager to get home. Entering from the passenger side meant that I needed to raise my left leg, the one that was just operated on. I found that raising my leg toward the truck was excruciating. I had to catch my breath and nearly fainted. I readjusted my stance and faced away from the side of the truck, lowered my hips back toward the seat, and had my partner and the nurse help me turn both legs together into the truck. The ride home was short, though every bump seemed to send shooting pains throughout my leg. I couldn't wait to get home, change back into my pajamas, and get into my own bed. I hope that by painting this picture you have an idea of how a simple task of maneuvering yourself into a vehicle for the ride home can be much more challenging than you expect.

You've shown great courage reaching this point. The worst is over and the healing has begun. You will either return home or receive additional care from a rehab facility. Welcome, you are now bionic and about to embark on a new adventure. Hang in there, you'll soon feel better and regain your independence.

CHAPTER 4
PAIN MANAGEMENT—BEFORE, DURING, AND AFTER SURGERY

There is only pain in resisting. Relax and yield.
—Stephen C. Paul (Illuminations: Visions for Change, Growth, and Self-Acceptance)

Describing and measuring pain is a challenging task for patients and medical providers. Managing pain is a priority when you have a chronic condition and become the new owner of an artificial joint. Minimizing your pain helps you gain quality sleep, keep your sanity, and improve your quality of life. Each and every one of us handles pain a little differently, experiences it differently, and will tolerate pain in differing degrees.

After surgery, you will experience the pain of recovery—incisions to mend, swelling to decrease, bruises that need to heal, and new and uncomfortable sensations as you adjust to the feeling of metal inside your body. Cold and damp weather may affect you and possibly create a "creaky" or "stiff" sensation. Plus, there may be internal pain near the tip of the metal implant in the middle of your femur. Joint pain tends to radiate out to surrounding joints as other areas of the body compensate for balance and strength. So our knees, ankles, and feet may also have their share of aches and pains. Each pain, ache, twinge, or sensation of discomfort is unique and might not respond to a one-size-fits-all treatment plan. You may already have a formula in place to handle your pain in regards to your joint. Whether you are pro medication or choose to tough it out, there are a number of pain management techniques to consider for relief.

The internal pain I refer to was a feeling I encountered during recovery. You might also notice this new sensation when you raise and move the affected leg—odd feelings from the head of the joint, along the hip and upper leg, to the implant tip midway in your femur. You may feel aches and strange sensations due to the metal components helping you move from the inside out. The feeling is a foreign one that is challenging to describe, though I'll do my best. A few weeks after surgery, I weaned myself from prescription pain medication and limited my dosing to right before bedtime. I didn't care for the side effects of the opiates, specifically the constipation and "dopey" feeling I had all day long. I decided I would rather feel some discomfort and opted to stop using the stronger pain medication. This time of heightened awareness is also when I began to notice the strange new sensation. It was icy cold, uncomfortable, and unnerving. I noticed it when I raised my leg, meaning the motion when you are lifting your knee toward the ceiling (a movement you'll make with knee lifts and leg raises taught during physical therapy). I felt this internal resistance halting my progress. The first time I noticed this feeling, I instinctively braced both sides of my leg a hand's width above the knee cap. I was concerned that I hurt myself. This feeling lingered and repeated with every similar movement.

My surgeon called this sensation "stem pain." The mechanics and placement of a new hip starts by placing it at the ball of the hip joint and inserting a metal shaft into your leg bone. The length of this metal stem and tip are where many patients have this sensation and sensitivity. If it sounds disturbing, it was and may be for you as well. Some people experience the feeling more than others; I describe it here for awareness and to allay any fears. I was assured by my medical team that the sensation would fade. Mostly it was a feeling that I became accustomed to as the bone healed and muscles strengthened. I chose to befriend this odd feeling and welcomed it—this internal titanium part was helping me to walk.

Both you and your surgeon will have a discussion about the types of pain medication that will suit your needs based on what you tolerate, medications that your doctor suggests, and what type of pain you are experiencing. Prior to surgery, I opted to avoid pain medication since my experience was one of feeling discomfort more than I actually felt pain. Stephen C. Paul's quote introducing this chapter is a reminder that pain can be managed, minimized, and even eliminated by any number of tools. Resisting is not an option; pain is part of this procedure. Music is one such tool; pain can vanish and become an afterthought as your mind is lost in a beautiful piece of music. There are many pain management tools that can help you, both medicinal and natural. Sometimes a variety of methods work best since the sensation of pain will vary during recovery. To manage my discomfort, I used multiple methods, detailed below.

ACUPUNCTURE

Receiving regular acupuncture treatments was by far the most effective remedy for me to manage pain and minimize my stress before surgery and as an ongoing practice afterward. Acupuncture also alleviated additional problems I had been dealing with such as lack of sleep, anxiety, and mild depression. Prior to this experience, I had never tried acupuncture simply because I mistakenly believed a person should have a medical need of some kind for it to be useful or applicable. I later learned I couldn't have been further from the truth. I had read about acupuncture, knew people who swore by the amazing results, and now understand the theories and mechanisms of why it works. Today I continue to be a regular client and can't imagine my life *without* acupuncture.

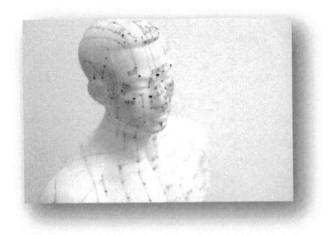

Acupuncture involves the placement of thin, single-use, stainless-steel pins (needles) at different areas of the body; the selection of the points on the body and the number of needles depend on the reason for your visit. Acupuncture has been practiced for thousands of years and has been gaining more acceptance in Western cultures for the past several decades due to an increasing body of evidence demonstrating its effectiveness.

To paint a picture for you: A typical appointment of mine starts with comfortable clothes. Sleeves and pant legs should easily roll up or be short enough to expose lower arms and lower legs. After checking in and choosing a recliner, the acupuncturist conducts a brief consultation to understand the reason behind the day's visit. Then, based on the conversation, needles are placed along the arms, legs, hands, feet, even scalp. Once all the needles are placed, the acupuncturist checks on my comfort and may cover me with a blanket. At that point, I close my eyes and take what is referred to as an "acu-nap." I feel immediate and long-lasting results.

Weekly appointments prior to surgery helped me avoid using anti-inflammatories, which were also hard on my stomach, and I slept much better. Within two weeks after surgery, I returned to weekly acupuncture visits and opted for table treatments in a private room instead of the communal room recliner. This enabled my acupuncturist to work much closer to the incision site. My surgeon was aware of and supported my decision to receive regular acupuncture for pain management.

A trained acupuncturist typically earns a minimum of a four-year degree, which includes an extensive education in pathology, anatomy, contraindications, dietary therapy, ethics, and more. Acupuncture is an ancient form of healing that predates recorded history. During the Shang dynasty around 1000 B.C. hieroglyphs portrayed acupuncture, and bronze needles have been excavated demonstrating the use of this treatment for centuries. Acupuncture is a historical medical treatment that, when performed by a trained professional, provides astounding health benefits with minimal side effects and will not counteract with other types of medical treatment or medication.

A word about finding a qualified, affordable acupuncture clinic—for my acupuncture treatments, I visit a community-based clinic where a number of people are treated at the same time in the same room. Community clinics focus on services that are accessible to all. Receiving your treatment in a room shared with others allows these clinics to offer acupuncture on a sliding scale fee. My acupuncturist belongs to a national cooperative called POCA (People's Organization of Community Acupuncture). There are over 200 cooperatives around the United States that participate following certain guidelines. One of these guidelines includes offering affordable treatments in a community setting. If you're in the Salt Lake City area, I recommend visiting the following website: www.qiworkscommunityacupuncture.com. For POCA locations in the United States, visit www.pocacoop.com.

Besides acupuncture, I also used prescription pain medication during my hospital stay and while recovering at home. During the first two weeks after surgery my use was minimal throughout the day—I would go as long as possible before taking another dose, at times breaking my pills in half, and preferred to use a full dose right before going to sleep. Talk to your doctor about which pain medication they suggest for you and understand the side effects. Using pain medication, I would sleep, though it definitely felt like a "drugged sleep" rather than a restful sleep—the morning after a dose of pain medication felt sluggish, heavy, and it took me an hour or so to feel clear-headed. Acupuncture was a wonderful option helping me to wean off the pain medication much sooner than my surgeon expected and didn't include any negative side effects.

PHARMACY

During the final hours of your hospital stay, you will receive physician orders as to which medications to continue taking in the days and weeks ahead. My surgeon advised me to continue blood thinners, antibiotics, and pain medication. Pain medication after hip replacement is necessary. This surgery invades tissue, tendons, and bone. Since everyone experiences and handles pain differently, the variety of pain medications available thankfully provide comfort and ease the aches and pain felt for weeks afterward.

When I arrived at the hospital pharmacy, I spoke to the pharmacist at length regarding the amount of pain medication I was being sent home with. I felt that 100 oxycodone tablets was a ridiculous and dangerous number since it is very addictive. I asked for half the amount with the ability to call my doctor for a refill and was surprised that my request was denied. I almost wish I would have taken 50 out of the bottle and left them on the counter. I live in a state where misuse and abuse of pain medications is high. Crimes such as home burglaries to get to medicine cabinets happen quite often. I begrudgingly took the full prescription, knowing I would never take this many pain pills. I fully intended to return a great deal of them for safe disposal in a few weeks once I was able to return to acupuncture and had time to rest and recover.

An unfortunate event happened that I hope you don't ever have to deal with. A person very near and dear to me betrayed my trust during my first week home from the hospital. They quietly and consistently broke into my pain medication. Pills were slowly stolen and used for addictive purposes. That indiscretion and the negative consequences that followed were tough to handle. My relationship with that person suffered greatly and eventually ended. Watching someone you love battle with any addiction is heartbreaking. With treatment and care, they can recover. However, relationships do not always mend from this experience.

I bring up this uncomfortable scenario to suggest caution when storing your medications. The temptation of such a powerful medicine can lead those with an addiction problem down a treacherous path. After my second and third surgery, I stored my medications in a secure space and asked my parents to keep the bottles at their home. When they visited, I would only keep a few days' worth safely stored. Sometimes a home health aide or nurse can supply you with a locked cabinet to keep all medications secure and out of harm's way. This is a good idea especially if you live in a busy household with young children, teens, or have frequent visitors. Protect yourself and those you care about, it's best to keep these potent drugs out of hands that shouldn't have access to them.

ARNICA

This homeopathic remedy continues to be a source of relief. Take a peek in my bathroom and you'll find a tube or two of this gel in my medicine cabinet. After surgery, arnica was part of my daily regimen—from placing the ingestible tablets under my tongue early on to topical treatment after the wound closed. I currently use both the gel and tablets to ease aches and pains along with any bruises I or anyone in my family inevitably winds up with during day-to-day living. This product is safe and works quickly for me. The gel applied to my low back in the evening helps to minimize any low back pain and arthritis aches that flare up during the cold winters we have in Utah. I occasionally work my way through a tube of the capsules if I have been active hiking or snowshoeing to recover from exertion and muscle aches. Arnica can be purchased in bulk, online, and at any number of big-box retailers to stock your medicine cabinet. Before using arnica, though, talk to your doctor.

ICE

The thought of cooler temperatures may not spring to mind when you are in pain. Ice is your friend and is much more effective than dry or wet heat for inflammation and pain relief. I certainly wouldn't dissuade you from soaking in a hot tub or mineral bath for comfort and relaxation when you are able, though to decrease swelling and quiet pain, ice is by far the preferred method. Ice packs should never rest directly on the skin. To avoid skin damage such as frostbite, always place a boundary, such as a towel or blanket, between your skin and an ice pack. Ice packs come in a variety of sizes and forms to treat large and small areas. Ice brings quick relief—the rule of thumb is to use ice packs for a maximum of five to 15 minutes.

Here are some affordable options that you may have in your home now:

- **Gel packs**—These can be reused and are typically rectangular; they also time themselves—once the gel pack is warm and soft it's time to place them back in the freezer for future use.
- **Frozen peas**—The small 10- or 12-ounce bags are a great size for the hips, low back, or knees and they can be reused. Once the peas begin to warm and soften, it's time to place the bag back in the freezer. Mark the bag with a permanent marker so you'll know that this bag isn't going to be the best for consumption.
- **Rice packs**—You can purchase these or, better yet, make them yourself with old tube socks partially filled with uncooked rice. Fill the tube sock loosely, so it feels like a bean bag, and tie off the end or sew it shut. The rice pack will retain cold temperatures well and the narrow shape of a tube sock is great for the low back or can be looped around your neck to relieve upper body aches. Store it inside a plastic bag in the freezer to prevent it from absorbing food odor. When you are ready to use it, remove it from the plastic bag, wrap with a dry towel, and place it on the area that needs pain relief. This type also slowly warms to body temperature and is great to use at naptime since it is nonperishable and soft.
- **Juice cans**—Mark the can with a permanent marker for therapy only and try these as foot rollers to alleviate any aches and pains you feel in your feet. Cans are also a great shape to place between your shoulder blade and spine to treat knots of tension in the shoulder muscles.

GUIDED IMAGERY AND MEDITATION

Meditation isn't mysterious. In fact, it's fairly simple once you begin to practice. You may have meditated already sitting quietly on your porch watching a sunset or relaxing in a cozy armchair. Meditation winds down an overstimulated mind. Our mind is a powerful tool. During meditation, brain waves move into a relaxed state. Guided imagery provides a script to direct your thoughts in a positive way. When you recall a pleasurable event such as a favorite vacation or a wonderful meal, how many senses are awakened in you? Can you picture the setting, evoke certain smells, and even recall vividly how something tasted? Both guided imagery and meditation harness your mind's abilities and can help with pain relief, stress management, and restorative sleep. Using these techniques for pain management is an affordable option. They have no side effects, co-pays, or restrictions, and with the use of a CD, download, or audio files, you can access them anywhere you have space to sit or lie down quietly.

I've already recommended the guided imagery title *Successful Surgery*, available at www.healthjourneys.com. Meditation is a similar method and can calm your mind as you focus on your breath. Meditation is a time to relax, settle down, and can take place anytime or anywhere. Walking meditations are a great introduction since you shift your focus on the act of walking, becoming more mindful of your movements, your breath, and the action itself. When you shift your awareness and focus only on a motion, your breath, or a thought, you lower your blood pressure, feel more calm, and most importantly, feel less pain. Meditating with a mantra—a sacred word or phrase—is a way to add a positive tone to your meditation time. Another element to add alongside a mantra is images. When you sit in meditation, chant a mantra, and hold your gaze on a beautiful visual, the experience can be quite euphoric.

A website I suggest is Jonathan Goldman's Temple of Sacred Sound (www.templeofsacredsound.com). Jonathan is a pioneer and authority on sound healing. Along with his website, he has authored numerous books and created over 25 award-winning recordings. The Temple of Sacred Sound website houses four toning chambers offering audio and a kaleidoscope of visuals. On the site, you choose one of the four tones then prepare yourself before entering the chamber. Once you've chosen a chamber, simply gaze at the medley of graphics and tone (chant) using the audio accompaniment as a guide.

EPSOM SALTS

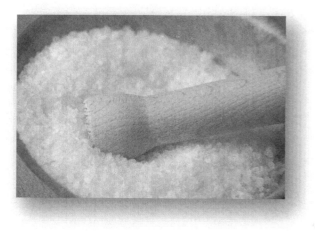

After your incision is fully closed and you are well enough to get in and out of a bath safely, try an Epsom salt bath. This affordable and natural aid is added to bath water or a small basin for a foot soak. Soaking in Epsom salts are restorative and leaves you feeling rejuvenated and relaxed. Epsom salts are basically magnesium sulfate and can be used both topically and internally—many people recognize Epsom salt as a laxative and aren't as familiar with the topical benefits. When it is dissolved in warm water, the magnesium sulfate is easily absorbed through the skin. Once absorbed, the cells use the mineral to relieve tension, energize the cells, and even increase serotonin. Epsom salts can also decrease inflammation. Epsom salts can be found in any grocery or drug store and are typically found near the foot products or laxatives. Package directions vary—for a foot soak, you can use one-half to one cup in a basin of warm water, and for a full bath use around two cups. Be cautious before you bathe with salts. If you have any small nicks or cuts, expect a stinging sensation during your soak. Laxative effects only apply if you drink a solution made with Epsom salts; soaking in them won't cause this effect.

A new discovery of mine was finding Epsom salts in gel form. I found a tube of ProCure Epsom Salt Rub and the gel form intrigued me. Since it allows spot treatment, there was no need to soak, and a tube is convenient for work, home, and travel. This particular brand included two additional ingredients that I favor—one is aloe vera gel and the second is my favorite homeopathic, arnica. I felt immediate results using this gel and the pain relief was long lasting. I've recommended this brand to others for arthritis pain, muscle aches, and joint pain.

MINERAL SPRINGS

Natural mineral pools are hydrotherapy provided by nature. One of my favorites is the world's largest hot spring pool located in Glenwood Springs, Colorado. Native Americans had used these sacred springs for many years, and in the late 1800s a public pool was constructed to harness the healing waters. Glenwood Springs was used as a convalescence home during WWII and has seen famous visitors such as Doc Holliday and President Teddy Roosevelt. Soaking in natural mineral springs provides me with an almost euphoric feeling. I leave feeling limber, no aches, no creaky joints, and no pain. Sleep after a mineral pool soak is some of the deepest, relaxing slumber I have ever experienced. I envy those who live near natural mineral pools. One of my goals is to hold annual retreats at a mineral pool with a group of people who have artificial joints—hips, knees, shoulders, the works! Wouldn't it be great to share stories and enter the water a bit stiff and achy and leave the pools as if you have just visited the Fountain of Youth? If you enjoy soaking in a warm to hot bath but haven't soaked in a mineral spring yet, add this to your bucket list.

According to the Glenwood Springs website, there are over 15 minerals in their pools, including sodium chloride, potassium sulfate, calcium sulfate, and calcium bicarbonate. These minerals, including the all-important magnesium, are often lacking in the human body and can be absorbed through the skin.

The Arthritis Foundation recommends soaking in mineral pools to ease pain, loosen joints, and manage musculoskeletal conditions. Soaking in these pools is a good place for physical therapy—the buoyancy takes pressure off the joints and water is a perfect partner for gentle forms of exercise. All of the exercises you learn during physical therapy are usually much easier in the pool. When you practice your fitness routine in a mineral pool, it's like exercise on steroids. You receive twice the benefit!

LAUGHTER THERAPY

Did you know that endorphins are released in your brain when you laugh and they act as natural painkillers? Laughter manages stress and minimizes pain. Humor is helpful in relieving tension and assisting you through long days when walking without assistance seems so far away. Make jokes when you have to put on those dreadful compression stockings. I pretended I was a saucy showgirl wearing thigh-high stockings to make my guy and I laugh while I wrestled them on and off. Watch a comedy, stream funny cat videos, whatever you need to lift your mood. Try www.patchadams.org.

Crying is another remedy that relieves stress. During an emotional cry, our body secretes chemicals in tears that are painkillers, which is why you tend to feel better after a long cry. Allow yourself to grieve and cry if you feel so inclined.

This is a crazy time that not many people experience. You are undergoing something completely new and learning to live differently. Those who receive an artificial joint do not "get better." We heal from the surgery, the incision closes, the bone will bond to the new equipment, and we become accustomed to a new way of living. Our health is forever compromised and requires ongoing maintenance and care. Seek gratitude to support you during this time of recovery and healing. Things are changing for you as the owner of an artificial joint, hopefully for the better.

CHAPTER 5
RECUPERATION—MILESTONES & TIMELINE

There's only one growth strategy: Work hard.
—William Hague

The time needed to recover from a hip replacement will vary from person to person. This variance is due to a number of reasons, such as level of health prior to surgery, the cause of your hip failure and need for hip replacement, your age, gender, fitness level, and whether your surgeon opts for a posterior or anterior placement of the new hip. Recovery time is also impacted by how well the surgery went, if you experienced any infections after surgery, physical therapy, and if other health problems are present.

Did you notice that some of these factors are under your control? Think patient power—you are in charge of your recovery and can make a huge impact on how well you heal. Even though there are unique components to each person's hip replacement recovery, it's beneficial to speak to others who have experienced joint replacements. This camaraderie can be helpful and even reassuring to learn what you are facing.

Many physicians expect patients to follow a general recovery timeline after hip replacement. I found it both discouraging and interesting that my experience with my first hip replacement on my left side was dramatically different from my hip replacement on my right side. We are all a little different, and even I had very unique experiences with all three of my surgeries. However, the guidelines below can give you an idea of what to expect. Understanding a variety of outcomes and hazards can help you prepare for your own recovery experience.

WEEKS 1 - 2

The early weeks of recovery after a hip replacement can be tough. It's also a time when you will see rapid improvement. The amount of time spent completing physical therapy exercises, getting adequate rest, and eating well will reward you with increased mobility and can speed the rate of healing. After returning home, the early weeks come with added demands such as home care to help change bandages and assess the health of the wound, blood draws to monitor blood thinners and aspirin, and physical therapy. Expect to increase your activity a little more each and every day with your isometric movements such as ankle pumps, leg swings, and walking, even if it is just around your home. You will tire easily and as few as eight to 12 leg exercises will feel difficult and demanding. Be gentle and use plenty of ice after exerting yourself to help with the aches and extra swelling created by movement. You may feel discouraged and that you should avoid movement, but consistent activity is crucial to heal well, promote circulation, and help you move forward in your recovery.

These first couple of weeks will give you an appreciation for anyone you have known with limited abilities. You may be in for a rude awakening, especially if you had a fairly active lifestyle prior to surgery. Getting out of bed, going to the bathroom, and dressing yourself is going to take extra time, care, and effort. Slow-paced living is how you are going to approach your day and your movements whether you like it or not. You do not want to dislocate your hip! For example, I never quite mastered the tool to help me put on compression hose and luckily had a significant other who could wrestle those stockings on and off for me. But even with help it took extra time. Recovery is going to be a time to relearn simple and complex tasks; the artificial joint has limitations on movements and abilities and while your bone, tendons, blood vessels, and nerves are mending, your actions will need to be methodical and well-thought-out.

In the hospital, your physical therapist will guide you on how to get in and out of your bed, sit and get back out of a chair or seat of a car, and how to handle stairways. Repeating what you learned and applying it at home will set up a new pattern and eventually become a habit. I use my upper body to support myself much more now than I had in the past and am accustomed to turning my whole body to get in and out of my car rather than the twisting motion I used in the past. My partner, who had always been a gentleman and opened doors for me, became increasingly aware of slippery floors, snowy walkways, and rugged terrain that might cause me to slip and fall. Written here, it may sound as if you will walk on eggshells and feel fearful. To a degree that is true in the early days when you are getting used to moving your new joint—pain and discomfort are great sources of feedback. You do not want to repeat this surgery. My goal is to take my current joints to the grave and, with good care, I can expect decades of use from my artificial hips.

Toward the end of week two, I felt quite well and since the surgery was on my left hip, I was able to drive and return to work. It felt wonderful to have that freedom returned to me. It's amazing how something as minor as driving down to my favorite coffee shop in the morning could feel so liberating. My first drive on my own also surprised me with a few challenges. The first being how anxious I felt at the thought of being in a car accident. My second challenge was arriving at the coffee shop, realizing there is no handicap entrance or an easy way to hold my purse using both crutches. Then, as I was standing at the counter I realized, "I am expecting myself to return to my car on crutches, with a purse, holding a cup of coffee." I felt like an impulsive ass that day, to put it bluntly. Hallelujah for the kindness and understanding of strangers who were watching my dilemma and helped me to my car. Silly me, I got ahead of myself that day after feeling confined and restricted. I didn't even consider that carrying a cup of hot liquid while on crutches is not a good idea. That is, of course, until I stood blankly at the counter feeling like a fool. For those brilliant folks who walk with these devices or use other equipment every day—I salute you and am forever humbled by this experience.

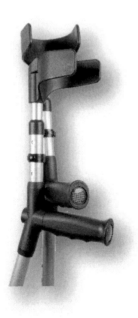

I chose the shorter crutches with all three of my surgeries and became more creative using them. I found the lower hand grip to be useful to help carry my purse and small grocery sacks so I could complete chores more easily. Any parent who has juggled a diaper bag, child, a stroller, purse, and grocery sacks gets fairly adept at using their behind, shoulder, and even forehead to open doors and get around.

On the topic of driving, once your surgeon gives the green light to drive again, you may want to apply for a temporary handicap license tag. You can typically find the required paperwork online from your local Division of Motor Vehicles, and your surgeon will need to sign it. The temporary tag is usually a minimal fee and will be dated based on the timeframe outlined by your physician. You must pick up this tag in person to demonstrate your ability, so there is no need to apply ahead of time.

Driving soon after a hip replacement means added health and safety risks. A sudden stop, running across a pothole in the road, or the smallest of accidents can cause injury and dislocation. Surgery on the right leg will take longer to heal and regain the strength needed to press the accelerator. Likewise, with vehicles using a clutch, the left leg may require extra healing time prior to driving. Understand your limitations. With either hip, your reaction time is slowed due to trauma, medication, and pain. Be cautious and access help running errands and commuting if needed.

If you do return to work after two weeks, remember to get up and move around every hour or two to increase circulation. Consider placing a footrest under your desk to raise your knees to hip level. This will help to reduce low back tension and support your hips. Take plenty of ice packs with you to manage discomfort. For those who have a lunchroom or cafeteria with access to ice, this might be fairly easy. Otherwise, instant ice packs found at the drugstore hold their temperature for 15 to 20 minutes and can help you make it through the workday.

WEEKS 3 - 6

During these weeks, you may find that you are moving with more ease, getting accustomed to your new routine and movements, and have freedom to shower. I speak from my own posterior placement experience; understand that those receiving anterior placement tend to heal more quickly. As your wound heals and muscles mend, you may transition from crutches to a cane or walking stick. Continue your physical therapy exercises, especially the leg lifts and leg swings. Realize that it can take six months to one year for the bone and muscles to fully recover from hip replacement surgery. Consistent exercise is crucial to help you return to an active life and protect you from dislocation. Walk often; this type of exercise is ideal. Your physical therapist will guide you toward the best treatment plan for your abilities.

I transitioned from crutches to a cane by week four and walked freely by week six (though I experienced a much slower recovery after my second hip replacement.) After my second hip, the right side, the ability to drive took a while longer since I needed the strength to press the accelerator. I returned to work after two weeks and arranged rides to and from work with family and friends. Unfortunately, I learned at week six that I had a fracture in my right femur, causing the implant to slip. This required a revision surgery. I stayed on crutches the entire six weeks after my second surgery, was scheduled for a revision at week eight, and continued for another 10 weeks until I could use a cane only. My muscle strength declined rapidly during my second surgery, so it took much longer to recover from the muscle atrophy and to regain my strength. The leg swings and isometric routines learned during physical therapy are exercises you should continue for the rest of your life to maintain muscle strength and tone. As my stories demonstrate, all hip replacement surgeries come with unique aspects of recovery and ability. Maintaining good lines of communication with your medical team and following their instructions is key to bouncing back from any setbacks.

You'll know that you can walk safely on your own without the support of crutches or a cane when you can stand on one leg without wobbling. Your surgeon may have you demonstrate this skill during a follow-up appointment. Do not try this balancing technique unsupervised. This is a great test during the early months of recovery to gauge your progress and notice how much stronger you become day after day.

One source of muscle and cardiovascular support during this timeframe of recovery is wearing the dreaded compression hose that I've mentioned. Many patients are able to stop wearing them about six weeks after surgery. I was very happy to throw these in the garbage, though oddly enough my first few nights sleeping without them did leave me feeling a bit vulnerable. The strength of healing muscles, mended blood vessels, practicing daily exercises, and staying well hydrated are the ongoing supports that replace the need for these stockings. Once you are able to stop wearing them, I'm guessing you won't miss them any more than I did.

Pain medication was essential to help me sleep during the first few weeks after surgery. The downfall to this reliance on medication was the heavy, achy, drugged state I felt after waking. This left me feeling incredibly sluggish in the morning. I am a morning person and wanted to return to my schedule of morning exercise, so that meant weaning myself away from the pain medication. As mentioned earlier, I minimized daytime use after week two, which enabled me to drive and return to work. Another uncomfortable side effect of pain medication is constipation. If you continue using the pain medication, consider adding stool softeners or laxatives to support regular bowel movements if you aren't using them already.

During weeks two, three, and four, I would occasionally take a pain pill after getting home from work and then one before bedtime. When I returned to work, I incorporated weekly acupuncture appointments to manage pain. By weeks five and six, I limited pain medication to bedtime only. I quit using the pain medication rather quickly in order to drive and to eliminate the negative side effects such as the "dopey" feeling and constipation. It isn't as if I was pain-free by any means during these weeks. I would rather feel a degree of discomfort than feel numb. Pain medication use is a very personal experience. Listen to your body, use your pain medication as directed, and speak to your doctor if you aren't feeling the relief you expect.

WEEK 7 - 3 MONTHS

This period of time is when you are able to walk on your own without crutches or a cane. Walk as much as possible from the beginning to regain muscle strength, mend, and build bone. Challenge your muscles and vary the duration of your walks. Exercise promotes bone growth that adheres to the new femoral cup in your hip socket. Choose ramps, inclined walkways, and slopes to improve balance and increase your cardiovascular health. Indoor walking on a treadmill is ideal for safety, convenience, and the ability to modify the incline and resistance as you progress.

As you wean yourself off pain medication, you will become more accustomed to the sensation of the artificial joint. I was acutely aware of the extra weight; the entire artificial joint weighs about one and half pounds. This may seem small, but try walking around holding a one pound weight in one hand only. After just a short time you feel lopsided and naturally want to switch hands to divide the weight. Of course, there is no switching with an implant, you just get used to it. Many hip replacement recipients notice something foreign is in their body. It takes some time to adjust to the feelings and be at ease rather than hesitating or stopping movements when you feel something strange. This is another reason I opted for less pain medication; I felt more aware of new sensations and could differentiate between pain, discomfort, and whether my body was simply getting accustomed to something new. Had I continued using pain medication heavily, I felt I was placing myself at risk of moving incorrectly and harming myself. As I regained my strength, I focused on adjusting to new feelings and making my movements fluid and smooth. This took time and practice. Understand that some hip replacement recipients elect to use pain medication much longer based on their tolerance and needs. There is no one-size-fits-all approach to decreasing pain medication. Do what is best for you.

INTIMACY

With a bit of hesitation and fumbled efforts, intimacy returned for us during this time period. Finding a comfortable position and reassuring my partner that he wasn't going to hurt me tended to dampen desire a bit. I felt self-conscious in regards to the appearance of my scar and sad that my movements were so limited. Lying on your side, kneeling, or standing is much more comfortable than the standard missionary position. This definitely isn't a sex manual and I'll trust that my readers are adults who know their bodies, their sexual expectations, and hopefully have a relationship that is open to negotiation. This is a challenging time. If you had a healthy sex life before your surgery, move forward with a sense of humor. With patience and experimentation your love life can return and be fulfilling. Your surgeon may not be the best resource if you are having challenges in this arena; a qualified sex therapist will be the most helpful.

SLEEP

As the swelling subsided, bruises healed, and muscles became stronger, the quality of my sleep also improved. I slept with fewer pillows under my torso and returned to lying flatter on the mattress during this timeframe. Gradually, I returned to one pillow under my head, one between my knees, and became a side sleeper. I do find myself alternating sides throughout the night to this day due to sensitivity around each scar. Resting a pillow between your knees while lying on your side prevents you from crossing your legs at night and maintains a position that supports the head of the femur in the hip socket. Rotating the knees too far inward or crossing your legs has an opposite effect and pulls the head of the femur away from the hip socket, which is a movement we want to avoid.

SUNSHINE

To encourage bone health, it is essential that you are receiving adequate calcium in your diet and enough vitamin D. Vitamin D is a fat-soluble vitamin that is stored in the liver. This important nutrient promotes calcium absorption. If you are deficient in vitamin D, bones can become weak and brittle. The problem with relying on supplements is toxicity due to over consumption. Also, vitamin D supplements may interact with medications such as steroids and cholesterol-lowering drugs.

Vitamin D is known as the sunshine vitamin since it is found in very few foods and is made internally when ultraviolet rays make contact with our skin. Research has suggested that five to 30 minutes of sun exposure between 10 a.m. and 3 p.m. at least twice a week to the face, arms, legs, or back lead to sufficient vitamin D synthesis.[4]

When I started walking without crutches and a cane, I spent more time walking outdoors to receive my weekly dose of sunshine. Sunshine is easily accessible, free, and can also boost your mood. This practice will help to mend your bone and support the new growth that will bond to the artificial joint. Spend moderate time in the sun every week. Our skin will never make too much vitamin D.

SELF-CARE AT WORK

Office workers, delivery drivers, or others who sit most of the workday may find that swelling and fatigue plague your work schedule. When I sat for more than an hour or two, my hips and lower legs would ache. A standing work station or incorporating a standing or walking break is a simple solution to support circulation and relieve pain. Remember that any long period of sitting places you at a higher risk for blood clots and also aggravates low back pain. To minimize my risk, I practiced my leg swings and lifts at work. During a break, it was easy to complete three sets of 12 in the handicap stall of the restroom. The larger bathroom stalls are convenient for privacy and provide added safety since grab bars are available. If you have an office or larger cubicle then set aside time for a leg-strengthening and stretching routine. Remember those ice packs! Instant ice packs are useful and convenient to manage any discomfort, swelling, and achiness. The disposable ice packs purchased from the pharmacy department are easy to use. Simply squeeze the bag—this starts a chemical reaction. Shake the bag to distribute the product evenly, and the bag cools quickly and provides 15 to 20 minutes of use.

SCAR CARE

Most of us already have a scar or two on our body. Even if you aren't bothered by the appearance of the deep scar after your hip replacement, caring for the scar eases any itching or tightness that you may feel. Scars differ in appearance and texture because they are fibrous and much denser than the skin they replace. A scar has no hair follicles and no sweat glands. The scarred area may appear stretched or puckered and be especially prone to dryness. There are a number of products and procedures on the market to improve the feeling and appearance of a scar; though they can be costly and include a number of risks. Expensive treatments such as chemical peels, injections, dermabrasion, and filler therapy have mixed results and may not be worth your while for a scar that will either be near the groin (for anterior hip replacement) or along the gluteal muscle (for posterior hip replacement). Vitamin E oil has been recommended, though some over-the-counter remedies have shown to be ineffective. Vitamin E oil has caused dermatitis and even worsened the appearance of scars in some cases.[5]

When you have a hip replacement, the scar may be only three to five inches in length, but it is a *very deep scar*. Deep scars reaching bone through muscle, tendon, and skin cause adhesions that limit movement and mobility. Per my doctor's recommendation, I used a product called Bio-Oil, massaging it into my scar morning and night using a technique called cross-fiber friction. Basically, you massage against the grain of the muscle in a circular motion helping to loosen, soften, and gently stretch the tissue. If you're a cook who prepares meat for the grill, you may have rubbed salt and spices into a roast or steak. The goal is to tenderize the meat by softening and stretching the tissue. Massaging your surgical scar is much the same, this technique can minimize the puckering and dimpled appearance as well. Even an older scar can benefit from this care. Our skin is living, breathing tissue made up of cells that regenerate daily. Massage sloughs off dead skin, brings blood and nutrients to the surface, and improves the health of our skin.

I applied Bio-Oil after bathing, placing a small drop or two (about the size of a dime) on my fingertips, massaging firmly in a circular motion across the scar. After a few weeks the scar began to flatten, the skin looked much smoother, and color of the scar lightened. Regular massage using the Bio-Oil helped to minimize the dimpling and puckered area on my right side since I had scar tissue within scar tissue due to my third revision surgery that reopened and lengthened the original scar.

Some may suggest using only a specific essential oil or moisturizing with vitamin A. Single ingredients may cause more harm than good, though. Bio-Oil, for instance, includes ingredients such as rosemary oil, chamomile oil, lavender oil, calendula oil, vitamin A, and vitamin E. Our skin is the largest organ of the body. Depending on the particulate matter, everything we place on our skin has the potential of being absorbed into the circulation. As outlined in an article on skin health, Dr. Thomas Campbell states that, "...in adults, there clearly are topical substances that cross the skin barrier. For example, medications applied to the skin can be absorbed systemically, and oils or other solvents can help facilitate their absorption." [6] This is why medications such as hormone therapy are available in patch form; our skin behaves like a sponge. The essential oils and vitamins in Bio-Oil are diluted, making them safer to use. Essential oils are very popular, very misunderstood, and often misused—these oils are concentrated and should be diluted in carrier oils before application. Some essential oils can adversely interact with medications and can also cause allergic reactions. Your pharmacist is a great resource to discuss concerns you may have about how medications and other healthcare products may react with one another.

While Bio-Oil has provided me with outstanding results, I have no doubt that the massage technique played a significant role. Since I am a massage therapist, I already take great care of my skin and know firsthand how much healthier skin will appear with regular massage treatments. When using any scar care product, do your research, talk with your doctor, and know that results come about only with consistency and daily use.

---

[4] Holick MF. Vitamin D deficiency. N Engl J Med. 2007; 357: 266–81.

[5] Shih R, et al. Review of over-the-counter topical scar treatment products. Plastic and Reconstructive Surgery. 2007; 119(3): 1091–5.

[6] Campbell T MD. I Avoid Eating Oil, but is it a Healthy Skin Care Product? T. Colin Campbell Center for Nutrition Studies. May 2, 2017.

CHAPTER 6
GOAL SETTING AND THE YEARS AHEAD

A goal properly set is halfway reached.
—Zig Ziglar

Goal setting provides you with a road map. In the beginning, after surgery, recovery may seem so far away. Your surgeon, physical therapist, and other medical providers are watching your progress and expecting you to regain strength and return to a more normal state at a certain pace. You should stay goal-oriented, helping to set an expectation of what lies ahead week by week or month by month.

MID-YEAR: 6 MONTHS POST-OP

The mid-year point in your recovery is a wonderful time. Crutches and canes are gathering dust in a closet, and you should be walking more confidently every day. There can be setbacks or complications that may hamper your success, such as a slip or fall or perhaps you aren't healing as quickly as you or your doctor expected. Where would you like to be in another six months? Set goals! Pay attention to X-ray results at your regular doctor visits. Are you mending as well as expected? Are you following your physical therapy orders and exercising as directed? How is your diet? Are you managing your inflammation as well as you possibly can? Hold yourself accountable. The success of your recovery and achieving your health goals is in your hands. Your surgeon, nurses, physical therapist, and other medical professionals can only do so much ... the rest is up to you.

Six months after my first hip replacement I changed careers. Illness and injury prior to learning that I required my first hip replacement led to my leaving a position as adjunct faculty and massage therapist at a local community college. Once I had recovered I sought employment with less physical demands and began working as a health and wellness coach. I was relieved to have a desk job since I felt that my days working in a physical profession were over. I was aware that sometime in the future I needed a second hip replacement. My new job, which provided health insurance, came at a perfect time in my life.

EMPLOYMENT

Discussing my hip replacement at work was uncomfortable for me. I am a private person and prefer to keep work and home separate. When it comes to medical situations and physical abilities, I prefer those conversations to remain between myself and my doctor. With this book, I've stretched my boundaries to share my health information and find that I speak much more openly about my artificial joints now. Depending on your line of work, you may never want to reveal that you have an artificial joint. If you are taking leave from a current employer and returning on crutches, you will naturally be questioned. Are you prepared for those conversations?

My second hip replacement and consequent revision surgery took place while I was employed. For the most part, the questions I received were of concern, mild curiosity, and care for my welfare. Unfortunately, there were also careless, nosy, and cruel coworkers who had no respect for my privacy. I experienced a period of hostility at the workplace. Manual labor jobs that require driving, lifting, twisting, and long periods in one place could be problematic or near impossible to return to. Your surgeon will discuss your employment prior to surgery and assess how you can return to work after recovery. Most employers are prepared to assist you with reasonable accommodations. Speak with your supervisor or human resources office if you feel you are experiencing any discrimination. Assert yourself and speak up for your rights. Ideally, your employer will work with you and want to resolve problems quickly.

Bending forward past 90 degrees will always be a no-no, specifically for those receiving a posterior hip replacement. Heavy lifting, anything over 25 pounds, is also discouraged. Excess exertion and specific movements may weaken pins in the femoral cap and can dislocate the joint. My surgeon provided me with a medical note outlining my abilities and limitations. Using this note, I was able to negotiate with my employer. After the human resources office granted an accommodation, my supervisor worked with me so I could keep my job. This process can take months and requires patience. Since hip replacements are not visible, they may be disregarded and thought of as "no big deal." You may encounter hostility and resentments. If you heal quickly, regain strength, and begin walking confidently, your coworkers may see you as "all better" and not needing accommodations. Living with artificial hips requires diligent care 24 hours a day, seven days a week. This is a balancing act as you gradually return to a more active lifestyle while you avoid treating yourself like a china doll. Live fully and enjoy your mobility, just be cautious. Dislocation, injury, or infection can send you right back to the hospital and the process starts all over again.

MASSAGE

This six-month landmark delivered a special bonus for me. I was *finally* able to lie face down comfortably and received a much-needed massage. While working as a massage therapist, I practiced what I preached and received monthly massages for over 17 years. I missed the relaxation, tension relief, and rejuvenation that a massage provides. I was surprised at how sore my quadriceps felt during the massage. My hips were so sensitive to touch that light pressure caused me to flinch. When tissue and nerve endings are cut, sensitivity is heightened. By continuing treatment with my massage therapist and practicing self-massage on my own at home, I increased flexibility, oxygenated the tissue, improved circulation, and promoted healing.

Invest in your health and incorporate regular massages into your routine. By regular, I mean at least one hour-long session every six to eight weeks. The health benefits within this time range have been well documented by pioneers in the field such as Dr. Tiffany Fields at the Touch Research Institute in Florida. Therapeutic massage offers an incredible amount of health benefits, including:

- Helps you manage stress
- Relieves tension
- Eases muscle aches
- Improves sleep
- Soothes anxiety and depression
- Lowers blood pressure
- Boosts immune function

Besides, a professional massage *feels wonderful!* Who doesn't want to feel better? Health insurance companies or health spending accounts may help cover the cost of a professional massage. Organizations such as the American Massage Therapy Association also offer a therapist-finder tool on their website, which is found at www.amtamassage.org/findamassage/find.html. Simply enter your zip code and search to read bios, specialties, and check credentials.

Many massage therapists specialize in a more clinical focus and have experience working with physicians, physical therapists, and chiropractors. Be aware that some states have different education requirements toward licensure. Massage therapists who have clinical experience typically have a higher level of education than many trade schools require. The massage industry lacks consistent regulation nationwide (meaning you don't always know the depth or scope of education the therapist has completed). You may not know if a massage therapist has fulfilled a minimal 100-hour training focusing on spa pampering techniques or has completed an extensive training equivalent to an associate's degree or higher. Your doctor may be able to refer you to a qualified massage therapist in your area.

AIR TRAVEL

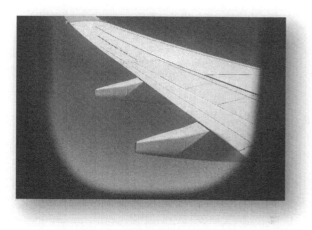

Allow yourself time to heal before planning any long trips. Speak to your doctor before you consider travel on an airplane. I chose to wait seven months before I made travel plans by air. While you are healing, air pressure changes experienced during flight and the immobility in a small cramped seat may cause your hip joint to swell. If you fly within six weeks after surgery, it is important to get up and move around during the flight and exercise while seated to encourage circulation. During the early weeks, you are at high risk for blood clots and remember, you will be wearing your compression hose. Practice simple exercises such as toe-tapping, knee lifts, and ankle rotations to improve circulation. These can be done easily on the plane without disturbing your seat mates. These exercises are also beneficial to practice on long car trips or any other time you sit for long periods.

When you fly, consider taking a medical alert card with you to show airport security. Before walking through the metal detector you may want to alert the screener about your artificial joint. Most major airports are prepared to accommodate customers with artificial joints and will screen you fairly quickly. Sometimes an additional pat down or extra security checks are required. Allow more time when you travel and notify the screener if you are in pain or if your hips are sensitive to touch.

1 YEAR

The first annual visit with your surgeon is an important one. At this appointment and subsequent follow-ups, X-rays determine the strength of your leg and hip bone, how well the femoral cup is adhering to the hip socket, and the overall placement of the new joint. If you haven't been receiving copies of your X-rays to take home with you, I suggest asking for them now. These are valuable records and help you better understand the importance of ongoing preventive health practices such as regular exercise, maintaining a sensible weight, and eating a quality diet.

Remember the checklist earlier in the book when you were planning for surgery? Continue to make a list of questions for the doctor and make the best use of your time and your physician's time. At this annual checkup you may be screened for arthritis (if you aren't living with this condition already) and given an update on the overall health of the surrounding joints. For goal setting, this one-year mark is a great accountability tool and will let you know how well you've been following doctor's orders and taking care of yourself. Ask your doctor if there are additional things you can be doing to improve your health. Most, if not all, of any surgery-related weight gain, should be eliminated at this point in time. If you are carrying excess weight, strive to reach a healthy weight for your body type. I realize this is hard work; weight loss takes determination and a great deal of effort. Want some added motivation? Managing a healthy weight increases the lifespan of your joint and may prevent you from a future joint replacement surgery.

SETBACKS

As I've mentioned, my second hip replacement took place 18 months after my first surgery. Unfortunately, I experienced some setbacks and didn't heal quite as well this time around. Due to a fracture found at the six-week follow-up appointment, I chose to have a revision surgery eight weeks after the second hip replacement. This was a tough decision to make. I knew I wasn't healing as well since I was still walking with both crutches at six weeks, unable to balance on one leg, and felt weak. Initially, I worried that it was my own cautious behavior that had slowed my progress. After my first hip replacement, and sensing that a second hip was in my future, I had been much more cautious during my physical therapy. I had also dramatically changed my workout routine to accommodate my new joint. When the fracture was found, the bone was already at the point of mending itself and, according to my surgeon, may have healed well enough to move forward.

Fractures can occur to anyone receiving hip replacement before, during, or after surgery. The bone is weakened, stressed, and at risk for failure. During surgery, your surgeon uses a mallet to drive the stem of the titanium replacement firmly into the center of the femur. My fracture may have occurred in the operating room, it may have happened during physical therapy, it may have shown up sometime during my six weeks of recovery. I will never know exactly when, where, or how my fracture came about. This fact doesn't concern me. Taking care of my leg and restoring it to the best state of health was first and foremost on my mind. One noticeable aspect of this fracture was that I limped due to one leg now being a bit shorter than the other. The fracture caused the stem to slip farther into my leg bone. I had two choices; the first was to avoid surgery and heal with a noticeable limp, accepting that a future surgery may be inevitable due to the weakness of the bone and limping movement compromising my health. The second choice was to prepare for a revision surgery as soon as possible to repair the fracture and reinforce the joint. The revision surgery would eliminate the limp and extend my recovery time an additional six to eight weeks.

I was alone at the surgeon's office when I was given this news and these two extreme choices. I sat calmly as I heard my options, looked over the X-rays, and stared blankly at my surgeon when he paused and looked closely at me. I realized later that I was in shock. My surgeon gently touched my knees and said, "You're taking this really well. How are you feeling, are you okay?" I felt dazed. When I left the office, my surgeon and I had agreed that I would determine within the week how we would proceed. My surgeon needed to adjust his schedule to fit in my surgery and I needed to speak to my employer and the insurance company. I sat in my car outside my surgeon's office that day and called my significant other first. As I told him what happened and what we needed to decide emotions took over. The severity and despair of this situation finally hit me. Between speaking to him, then calling my mom, and calling my boss to let her know I would be late returning to the office I sobbed and sobbed. The thought of going through another hip replacement surgery, all over again, was heartbreaking. A revision surgery is a more aggressive surgery that cuts into the existing scar, adds more metal, and requires additional weeks on crutches, wearing the compression hose, and basically feeling like hell.

I elected to have the revision surgery. After weighing the pros and cons, speaking to family and my employer, I decided this was the best option for me. I was able to take a leave of absence from my job using family and medical leave since I had exhausted my sick leave already after the recent surgery. Thankfully, my insurance company approved the procedure and covered a portion of the cost of surgery. In less than a week after learning about the fracture, I was scheduled again for surgery. I began my steps for preparation, recovery, and healing all over again. Due to the revision, I spent 18 weeks on crutches that led to significant muscle atrophy on my right leg (from the second/third surgery) versus the left leg (the first hip replacement). Revision surgery is extensive and, depending on the reason for the revision, you may receive added hardware and a larger incision. A second surgery that enters a fresh wound also increases the risk for infection.

Revisions are rare, and I hope that you will not experience this type of surgery. I urge you to pay attention to your body after surgery. Don't hesitate to call your doctor's office and ask questions if you see or feel something that seems odd or out of place. Problems may show up at any time after a hip replacement. For example, about six months after my revision surgery I noticed a slight depression in the center of my upper right thigh. This depression was nearly half of an inch deep and about an inch long. It literally looked as though someone had taken a small ice cream scoop and removed a half circle of tissue on my thigh. I didn't feel any pain, this depression truly showed up overnight. That was a creepy visual!

I scheduled an appointment at my surgeon's office and both my doctor and physician assistant surmised that nerves in my leg must have been damaged due to the metal bands placed around my leg bone during surgery to help mend the fracture. My physician assistant provided a solution: that I modify my exercise routine by adding additional leg swings and spending time on the treadmill at a higher incline to challenge the area. The muscle strengthened and the depression I saw went away (though it has shown up to a smaller degree when I slack off on my exercise routine).

Anyone who has experienced a limb set in a cast knows how quickly muscle can weaken. Use it or lose it applies to us all! Due to my lopsided living and weakness on the right side I had a lot of catching up to do. After I could walk without crutches it took nearly a year to strengthen my leg muscles so that both legs were the same size. It was hard work and kicked my ass to the curb.

Setting goals to pursue an active lifestyle and care for this bionic body has motivated me nonstop. I am grateful that I had terrific caregivers at my doctor's office that supported me completely.

2 - 3 YEARS

Once you've become accustomed to your hip replacement and have stepped past the one-year mark, you'll notice remarkable changes.

Nearing year two and beyond, movements seemed much more natural, flexibility increased dramatically, and my confidence to take on more aggressive activities returned.

I began hiking, not just a small trail; I took on strenuous hikes through Bryce Canyon and Zions National Park. There were a few moments on steep inclines that I felt pushed and took many more stretch and rest breaks than in the past, but I did it and it felt amazing. Wouldn't it be terrific if a group of artificial joint recipients could hit the trails together? I know I would love that! Your surgeon may have or know of a support group in your area that is interested in sharing activities. Or start your own.

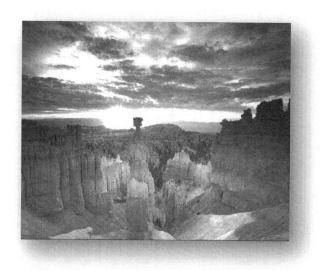

I snowshoed through fairly deep powder for one to two hours and felt invigorated. My time spent strengthening my legs and focusing on balance exercises paid off. I did feel a little nervous along hillsides and at steeper angles. Slow and steady wins the race, as long as I take my time and pay attention to my footing I snowshoe really well. I took it easy on the golf course since the twisting and rotation motions made me feel a bit uneasy. I warmed up before a round and stretched continually, as anyone should before activity. I've met other hip replacement recipients who are braver than me and returned to the ski slopes. I opted out of skiing since I wasn't a strong skier beforehand. Dancing and hiking are the activities that I placed the most importance on. My dance moves aren't quite as sassy and smooth as in my younger days, but I can still shake my groove thing with the best of them.

What activities and movements are on your wish list? Are you participating in the exercises and stretches that support you and ensure that you have the strength and ability that you desire? Besides regular strength training, walking outdoors and on the treadmill, I incorporate regular stretching and isometric exercises. My fitness routine isn't overly strenuous. The most important aspect is that my fitness routine is regular. I've found that daily exercise, for 30 to 60 minutes, allows me to feel my best.

4 - 5 YEARS

Prior to becoming ill, I was flexible and able to sit cross-legged, not exactly a full lotus position, but I sat this way comfortably and with ease. Moving your legs outward, away from the body, is a safe movement. Bringing your legs across the body, toward the center, or even crossing your legs while seated are dangerous movements and should be avoided. Sitting cross-legged, knees outward, is a more advanced movement. This seated position was a rotation that I eased into gently. Four years after my first hip replacement, three years after the revision surgery, I vacationed at Glenwood Springs to soak in the mineral pools I introduced you to in Chapter 4. After a long day soaking and relaxing, I returned to the hotel room feeling invigorated and limber. I surprised myself and my significant other when I instinctively sat on the bed—cross-legged—with my knees *comfortably* resting on the mattress! We had been laughing and talking when I walked into the room and basically plopped into that position smoothly and with no thought. What a thrilling feeling to have, and it came about easily and naturally! This was an achievement in freedom that I had longed for. After years of cautiousness and fearing what not to do, I had found myself spending too much time over-thinking my motions and slowed myself down when I didn't always need to. I felt no hesitation in this movement while on vacation and my reaction that day felt more normal than my activity had been for quite some time. It was a bit amusing as I eased *out* of the position; I wasn't quite as confident to quickly straighten my legs and get off the bed. Time will liberate you to move more freely and with more ease.

Rules and contraindications apply to us bionic kids with a posterior placement, specifically the no bending forward past 90 degrees and avoid lifting items over 25 pounds. These remain on the no-no list. I received that warning as a wake-up call at my two-year follow-up appointment. I still worked for the health insurance company at the time and traveled a great deal for work conducting benefit fairs and assisting the health team with biometric screenings. For these trips, fairly large bins holding our equipment were carried onto the site. The force of the lifting, even of bins weighing less than 25 pounds, placed enough pressure on my lower back and pelvis that the cup and screws of the femoral head were lifting *away* from my pelvic bone. That was horrifying news! My surgeon provided me with another medical note and, after negotiation with my employer, I was given help to avoid excessive day-to-day lifting.

Just another reason to pay attention to your body, schedule regular checkups and X-rays from your surgeon, and take care of yourself. There are days when I feel so incredibly creaky that I lie on my back and draw my knees to my chest just to put on shoes and socks. Other days, these tasks are handled easily. Bending to reach our feet is tough and drawing your knees up may be a movement you never regain; a long-handled shoe horn and slip-on shoes with Velcro closures may be a more suitable choice. Winter is tough for me. Cold days, especially those below freezing, leave me feeling stiff. I layer with insulated clothing and, even though I dislike them, I wear pantyhose occasionally for added support. Even years after surgery, modifications and adjustments are needed to maintain a good relationship with your bionic parts.

FALL PREVENTION

Throughout your recovery and long afterward, physical therapy, exercise, and weight management not only maintain health and fitness. These practices prevent falls. Exercise that encourage balance, home modification, and learning to move safely are all routines that will keep you upright. Falling is serious when you have an artificial joint. Falls may mean dislocation.

My first fall took place at work during the summer of 2015. As you read the scenario, see if you notice the mistakes I made. At the time, I worked on the fifth floor of a downtown building. My position required that I walk from our five-story building on a regular basis and visit our two sister buildings across the street for supplies, company vehicles, the copy center, and to attend meetings. The day I fell was a dry summer day. I was wearing flat gladiator-style sandals that were secure at the heel and had a fair amount of tread. I regularly took the stairs for exercise and this day was no different. I was carrying a few items, but they weren't heavy nor did they obstruct my view. Walking up a stairwell, I reached the fifth floor and hurried around a corner. The front of my sandal caught the step and I fell forward, striking my shin along the lip of the concrete step.

I caught myself, items scattered down toward the fourth-floor stairwell and I huddled in shock for a long time. My shin was bleeding and I didn't dare move, fearing that I had harmed my hips. Thankfully, my hips were okay. The gash on my shin left a horrid scar and I learned a valuable lesson.

Did you notice the mistakes I made? First, I was in a hurry. Second, the shoes that I wore that day led to this fall. Even though they were flat, wrapped firmly around the back of my foot and were sturdy, the front flap of the sandal lifted from my toes as I walked. Those sandals were a hazard destined for the trash. Lastly, I walked up a steep stairwell carrying items that prevented me from being able to hold the handrail. This event was a valuable and painful lesson. Modifications to prevent this scenario from happening again were fairly simple: Use the elevator when my arms and hands are full, always wear safe footwear, practice better time management so I'm not in a hurry, and don't be too proud to ask for help!

An interesting opportunity arose with my current employer in regards to falls. I now work as a health educator for a local health department. Part of my role is to focus on injury prevention within the community. I am certified as a falls prevention specialist and trained to teach an evidence-based program called Stepping On. I felt it ironic, appropriate, and as if synchronicity was at play when my supervisor informed me of this opportunity. Who better to teach this course than someone who focuses daily on preventing a fall? Stepping On is taught in many states across the US at community centers, hospitals, or in senior centers. You can learn more about Stepping On, and find a workshop near you, at the following website: www.wihealthyaging.org/national-stepping-on_1.

YEAR 5 AND BEYOND

The two most powerful warriors are patience and time.
—Leo Tolstoy (War and Peace)

I had been told by my surgeon and other hip replacement recipients that year five was the magic number. I didn't know if this was urban legend or simply a hopeful promise to keep my spirits up. Supposedly this post-five-year period would begin a timeframe that I would feel my best. Holy smokes, they were right. Five years after my first hip replacement I felt that my movements were fairly smooth and unencumbered. I don't know if this was placebo effect or not. At year five and ever since, I wouldn't just have good days, I had good *months*, and good *seasons*. My body, actions, and abilities behaved much more like what I remembered from my healthy preoperative joints.

In the days, weeks, months, and years that follow your hip replacement, you will find new routines, smoother movements, and an ease as you make peace with the equipment inside of you. You may feel creaky, grumpy, and stiff during the winter months. You may feel strange aches, take a bit longer to get out of bed in the morning, you will have lost those great dance moves you once had (they may have faltered in time anyway), and you will have interesting moments in the airport with TSA representatives.

I do miss my natural joints—you may or may not share that thought, but I still grieve the days when my legs were leaner, and my hips were scar-free. Acknowledge whatever you feel, whether it is anger, fear, relief, apprehension, shock, disbelief, and perhaps even joy. A hip replacement may restore you to an ability you never had before. Perhaps you are the person who will walk without a limp, with less pain, and straighter than you've ever walked before. This procedure is amazing and I'm grateful that the technology is available to provide us with years of mobility and movement.

Connect with me online if you'd like an extra source of support, I wrote this book and created my website to help others who are healing from hip replacements. We needn't travel this bionic path alone.

CHAPTER 7
FINAL THOUGHTS: BEYOND
SURVIVING, *THRIVING*!

My mission in life is not merely to survive, but to thrive;
and to do so with some passion, some compassion, some
humor, and some style.
—*Maya Angelou*

Do you recall watching old football commercials asking the quarterback what they planned on doing after winning the Super Bowl? Their smiling reply to the camera was, "I'm going to Disneyland." I couldn't agree more!

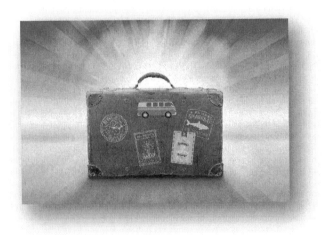

A trip to Disneyland was the first sizable reward I gave myself after my first hip replacement. My surgery took place in January and I spent four days at Disneyland the following August. Growing up with a grandmother who lived in southern California meant that I visited Disneyland regularly since I was six years old. I'm currently

52 years old and have visited Disneyland at least 35 times. If I lived near enough, I would probably visit weekly. After a recent trip, though, I decided that I can no longer ride the Matterhorn Bobsleds. The jostling and twisting motion of the carriage left me feeling incredibly sore. I have always loved riding the Matterhorn, but an injury isn't worth the risk. I'll enjoy from the ground.

Thriving for me means that I am enjoying my life to the fullest. When I learned that I needed a joint replacement, my initial fears were that my lifestyle would diminish and that I would lose physical freedoms. Prior to surgery, I didn't know what to expect and what I may never get to enjoy again. These fears and apprehensions are typical when we face the unknown. I knew that my life would change as I aged. Slowing down and losing physical abilities is fairly natural. I also believed that would be when I was in my 70s or 80s, not my mid-40s. Experiencing a health crisis leading to hip replacement at age 45 put me in a state of shock. I envisioned the possibilities of my future collapsing. Instead, this experience has been humbling and given me an opportunity to focus on what I can do. Today, I pay more attention to my body, my movements, and am aware of my surroundings. I scan ahead while walking to avoid slipping hazards, I wear solid shoes with nonslip tread, and follow a sensible fitness routine to stay lean and strong.

Breathing life into this guide and starting a new professional chapter has heightened my feelings of renewal, growth, and helped me grieve what I felt I lost. There were days I wanted to run away and just give up. Those feelings never lingered long. After all, where could I run? Change is inevitable and, like it or not, I had a new body to care for and a new lifestyle to embrace. Learning to live with chronic conditions and embracing new mechanical parts have changed me and my lifestyle. It will change yours as well.

This is a modification, simply something about you that requires careful attention and diligence. A person with artificial joints has a high-maintenance body—we all do, really. By investing in yourself with quality food, rest, and exercise you set the stage for many healthy years ahead. I see my body as my soul's vehicle. I care for my body, my organic vehicle, as I care for my car. I drive a Chevy Cavalier that has taken me over 180,000 miles since 2004. I plan on many more road trips with both my physical body and my Cavalier. My bionic buddies are my partners in this venture. I plan on my artificial joints driving me around for at least a few more decades taking trips to Disneyland, exploring hiking trails, and gliding across the dance floor. My surgeon informed me that with good care I can easily expect 25 to 30 years of use from my artificial joints. It's nice to have an idea of an expiration date. Around three decades provides me with plenty of time to live and play. What will I do if I face future surgeries? I'll cross that bridge if it presents itself.

Traveling to a theme park like Disneyland or visiting an amusement park may not be your cup of tea. Whatever activity you enjoy, hobbies that inspire you, or interests that motivate you, discuss them with your doctor and physical therapist. Medical professionals need to have an understanding of you and your lifestyle. A quality physician and their team will care about these aspects of you. Their job is to do their best to restore you to a level of health so you can enjoy what you love. Your job is to take steps daily to maintain your strength, stamina, and ability to hike, bike, golf, dance, whatever activity you wish to participate in! You are in charge of making those desires a reality.

This brings me to the present and the closing of this book. As I wrote these chapters, I also worked with a web consultant to create a website that would house, promote, market, and sell my book. The foundation of the website is to offer free resources and create a space where hip replacement recipients and others managing chronic conditions can connect and find support. I enjoy meeting others who are living with artificial joints. It's a bit like meeting friends and colleagues to share stories, discuss our experiences and triumphs, and console one another over what we may still miss.

Contact me online and join my tribe by paying a visit to www.andersontherapeutics.com, a virtual space supporting people who are managing chronic health conditions. Share your experience with me; I would love to hear from you. Register online and subscribe to my *Thirsty Thursday* wellness blog, consider joining me during one of my quarterly Goddess Retreats, or sign up for health coaching services. Partner with me to live well and be well.

Yours in health,

Tiffany

ABOUT THE AUTHOR

Tiffany Anderson is a health educator, alternative healthcare practitioner, writer, and health coach. She specializes in managing chronic disease, stress management, and pain management. She has worked in the field of health since 1996 and believes in practicing what she preaches by eating well, exercising daily, and investing in self-care methods such as receiving regular massage, Reiki, acupuncture, and practicing meditation. A Utah native, Tiffany enjoys hikes both locally and in the national parks, playing golf, dancing, gambling on occasion, listening to live music, and visiting Disneyland as often as possible. Her parents are retired and are two of her favorite travel companions. Tiffany is an empty-nester and has one grown son, Damien, and one beautiful grand-kitty named Dax. Readers can connect with Tiffany online at www.andersontherapeutics.com.

ABOUT THE PUBLISHER

Glass Spider Publishing is a hybrid micropublisher located in Ogden, Utah. The company was founded in 2016 by writer Vince Font to help authors get their works into shape, into print, and into distribution. Visit www.glassspiderpublishing.com to learn more.

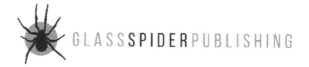

Made in the USA
San Bernardino, CA
09 November 2017